Close your eyes,

take a breath,

slow down

and return to a path

you never left

PLANT SPIRIT MEDICINE

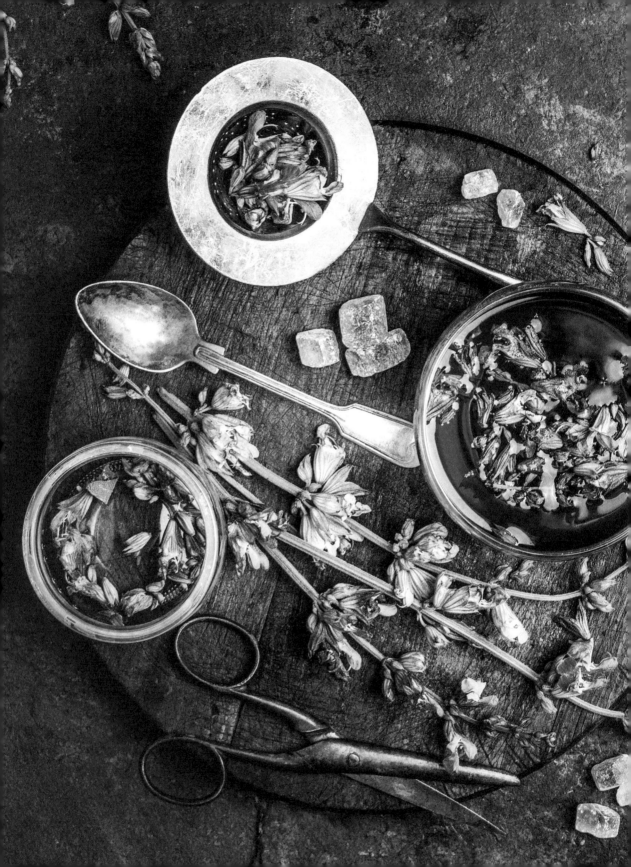

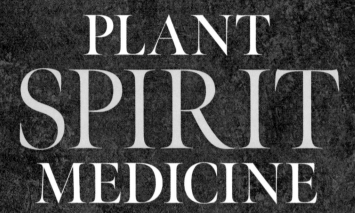

PLANT
SPIRIT
MEDICINE

A GUIDE TO MAKING HEALING
PRODUCTS FROM NATURE

NICOLA McINTOSH

ROCKPOOL

A Rockpool book
PO Box 252
Summer Hill
NSW 2130
Australia

rockpoolpublishing.com
Follow us! f ⊙ rockpoolpublishing
Tag your images with #rockpoolpublishing

ISBN: 9781925924732

Published in 2022 by Rockpool Publishing

The information in this book is not intended as medical advice. Check with your health practitioner before using any plant material for medicinal purposes.

A catalogue record for this book is available from the National Library of Australia

Printed and bound in China
10 9 8 7 6 5 4 3 2

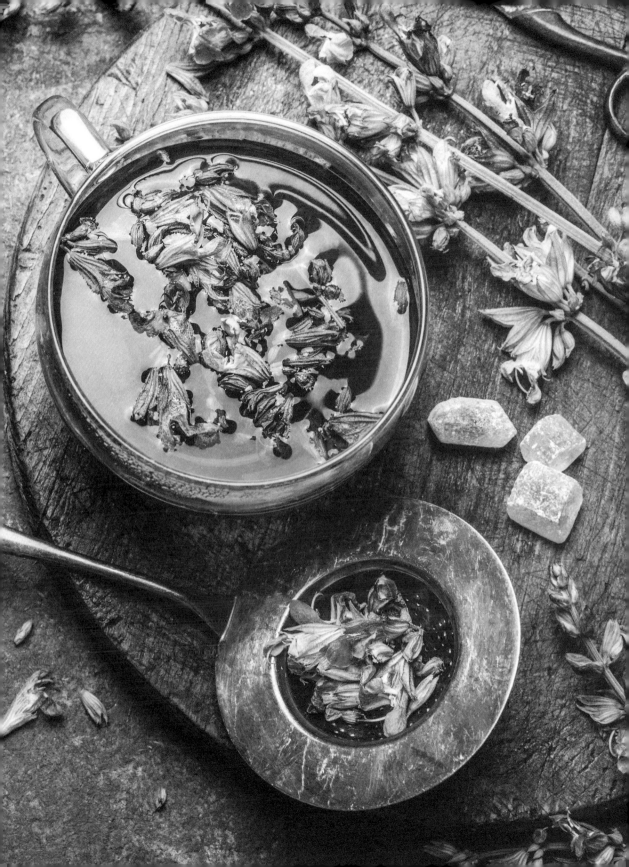

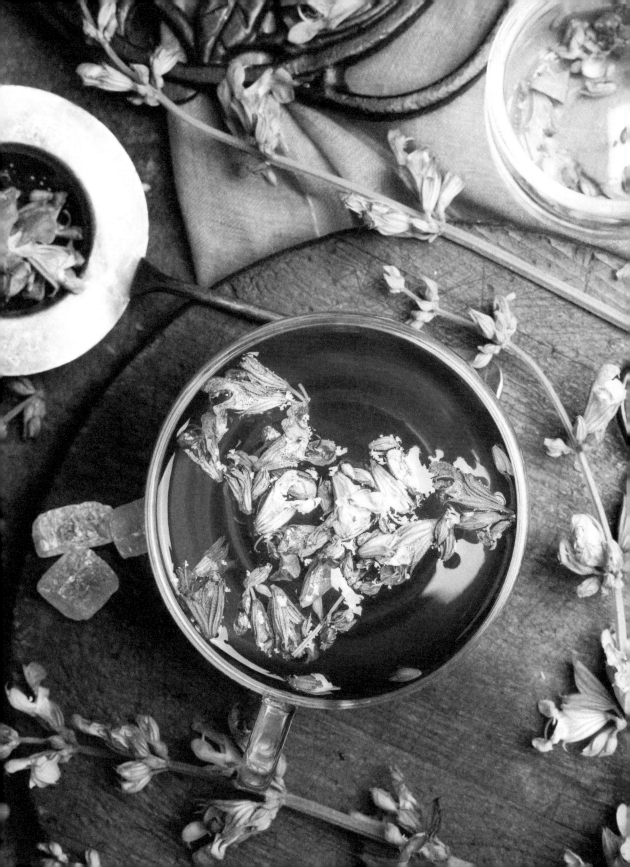

Dedication

To all who wish to find a deeper connection with nature and themselves. Walk the path with respect, gratitude and an open heart.

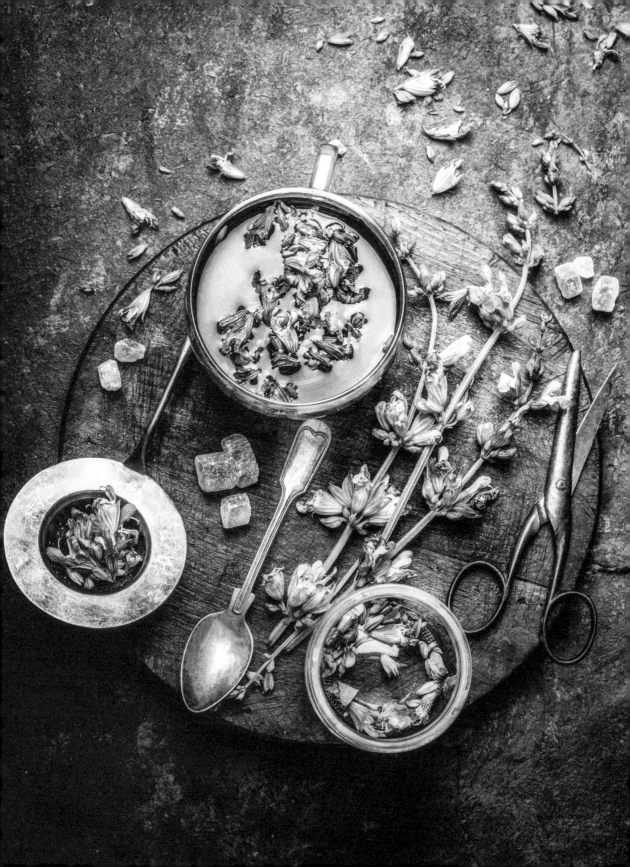

Contents

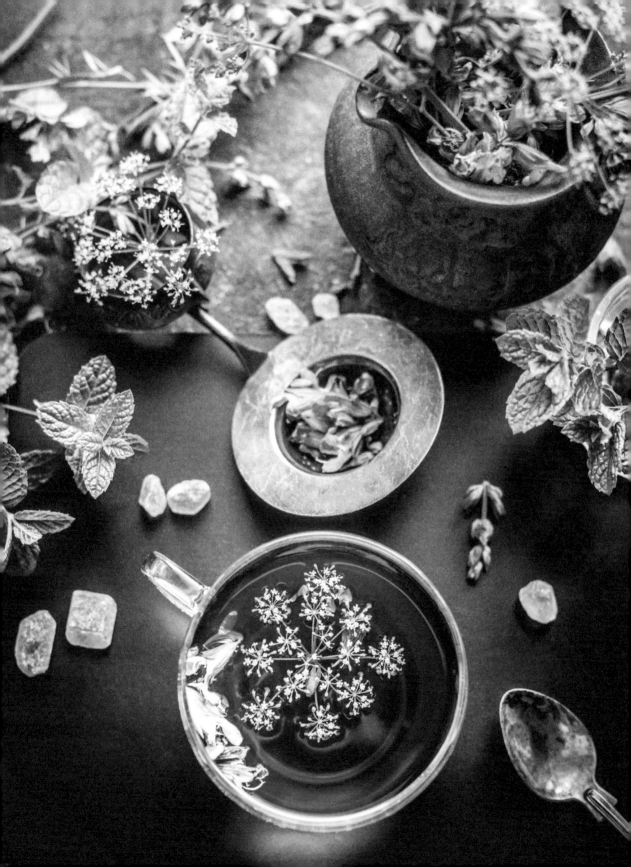

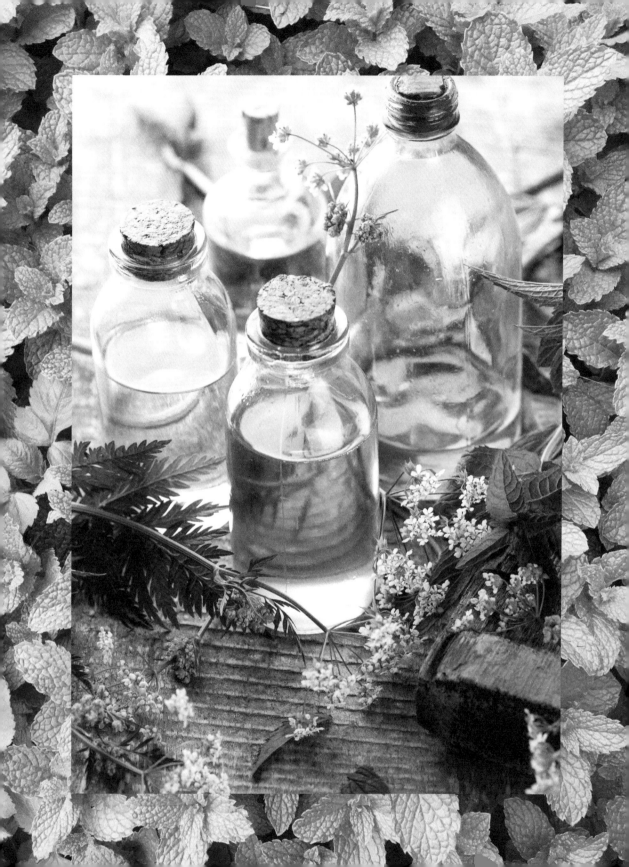

Preface

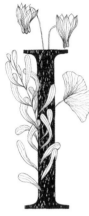

I f you have found my book, you – like me – are most likely a herb-nerd/ enthusiast, spiritual practitioner or environmentally conscious spirit. Welcome. This book is for both the beginner and the more advanced, and I have tried to cover as much as I can to encompass all levels. It not only explains in detail how to create wonderful natural products you can use for yourself or friends and family, it also provides a holistic view of working with the plant spirit – in itself, a potent medicine that works on the emotional and spiritual aspects of ourselves. Indigenous peoples from all around the world have worked with plant spirits for thousands of years, and this is how they came to know what specific plants were used for.

There are many books already published on Plant Spirit Medicine that go into detail on how to connect with different plants and the theory behind it. This book is about exploring the 'making' side of things. I suggest you read some of the many wonderful books on this subject to help you learn about Plant Spirit Medicine more wholly. I recommend *Sacred Plant Medicine* by Stephen Harrod Buhner, who also wrote *The Secret Teachings of Plants* and *The Lost Language of Plants*. Other books I recommend are *Plant Spirit Shamanism* by Ross Heaven and Howard G. Charing, *Plant Spirit Healing* by Pam Montgomery, and *Sacred Plant Initiations* by Carole Guyett.

I would ask you to do your own research where you can, experiment often until the processes become familiar and don't take shortcuts. If you are time poor, don't try and cram your practice into a small time slot. Make some time when you can immerse yourself into the work. Take time out of your routine, make a cuppa, slow down and give this your attention. Nature isn't out there racing, and to connect to it we need to be in alignment with it. As with any relationship, it takes time to get to know one another and it requires you to listen well.

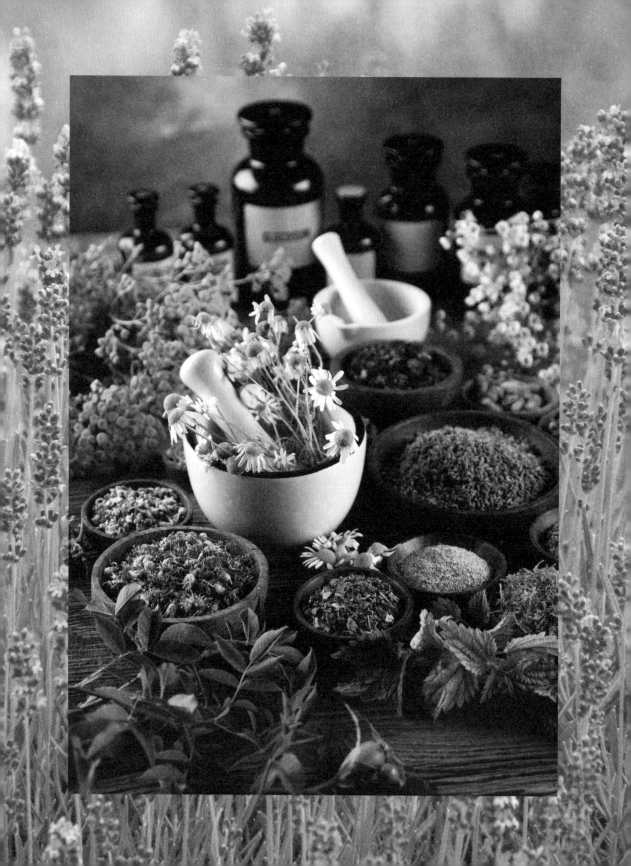

CHAPTER 1

Plant Spirit Medicine

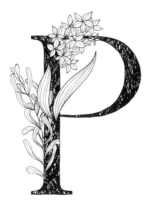

lant Spirit Medicine. What is it? Why do we need it? How can it help me? All valid questions in this day and age. Our Western society has grown accustomed to quick fixes – drugs, painkillers to help us keep going despite the pain, cold and flu drugs to push us through our colds instead of resting. We've all done it – we've all had to at some stage. We have to keep pushing through to make money to put a roof over our head and food on the table. The world is travelling at such a speed, it feels like we are going to hit the wall soon, and for many of us, that time has already come. We are exhausted; we are depleted; we are losing stamina, motivation and hope at times. Many of us are becoming increasingly unwell, and this is not only from constant stress, poor diet and a sedentary life, but also from our disconnect to the natural world around us.

Our modern world has created such stressors and separation from the natural world that we have become spiritually malnourished. This lack of attending to our spirit's needs is creating dis-ease on a mass scale. We are so busy looking at how to fix our physical body that we are not spending enough time looking at what our spirit needs.

We have isolated ourselves from that which should be sustaining us physically, emotionally and spiritually. We are searching for meaning and wanting to look after ourselves better. We are dealing with traumas in our lives, while still needing to soldier on. These are the issues that can stop us from getting better. There is no magic pharmaceutical pill for these kind of issues.

Obviously not all of us feel like this, not all of us are in search of medicine at this time. For those who are, Plant Spirit Medicine can help heal the parts of our soul and psyche that is so desperately needed at this time.

Having trained in both Western Herbal Medicine and Traditional Chinese Herbal Medicine, I felt one essential piece was completely overlooked in my training – working with the plant spirit. In fact, working with the physical plant, full stop.

When I had finished my Western Herbal Medicine degree, I knew the properties of the herbs inside and out and how to treat many conditions effectively, yet if I were to walk through an actual herb garden, I wouldn't be able to point out more than a handful of herbs. Our learning was all on paper and the herbs we used came as tinctures – herbal liquids in brown bottles. Sometimes we are referred to as the brown-bottle herbalists. We didn't gather our own herbs; we didn't get to know the herbs and their cycles.

The same can be said for my Chinese Herbal Medicine degree, although we did work more closely with the dried herb in many dispensaries, and these were the days I cherished in clinic. I came alive when I walked in the door. I could feel, smell and see the herbs everywhere. I tasted them, I handled them, and I just wanted to make things with them. I always put my hand up

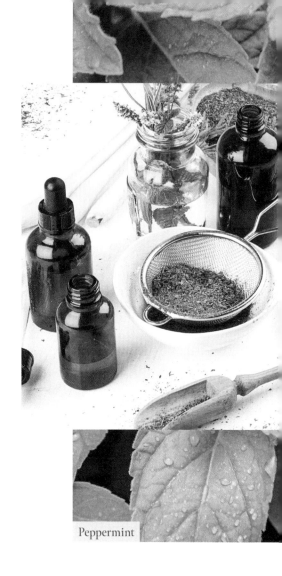

Peppermint

I would leave at the end of the day with herb dust in my hair and up my nose – and I felt great!

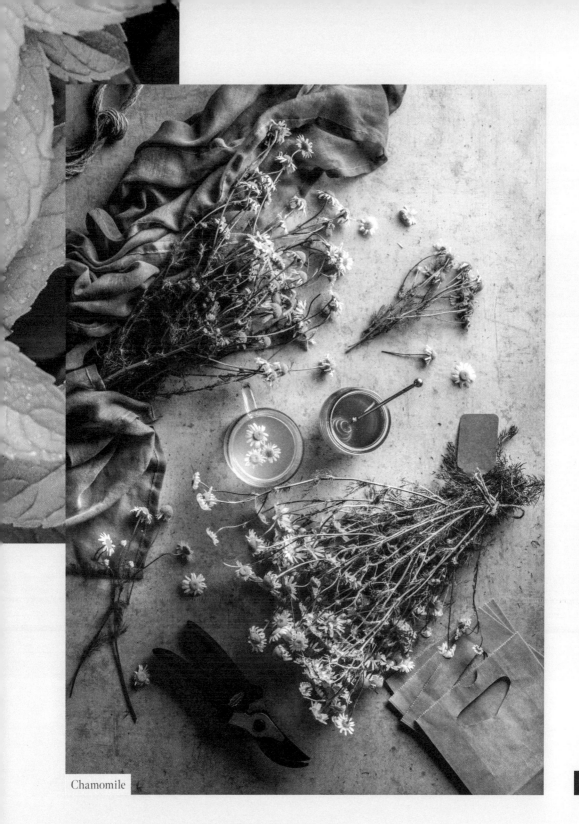

Chamomile

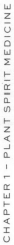

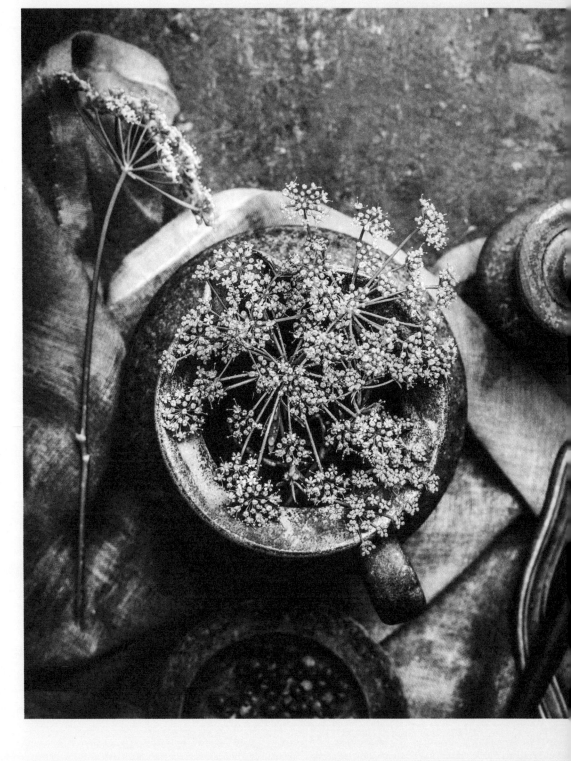

to do all the herb grinding to make powders, and I would leave at the end of the day with herb dust in my hair and up my nose – and I felt great! Other clinics, however, only stocked herb pills and powdered herbs in plastic bottles.

Now don't get me wrong – all these methods of herbal treatment still work, and I've seen incredible results in patients that doctors have had no success with. I don't get on the bandwagon of taking sides of herbalists vs doctors either. Each have their place and one must always seek out the treatment that works for them. In the hospitals in China, the doctors are dual trained in western and eastern medicine. I did a three-week internship in a hospital in Nanjing. It was incredible to see the whole hospital use both pharmaceuticals, herbs and acupuncture if required. It was all about what the patient needed and what worked the most effectively, and there was no contest between which was better.

One thing I did notice in clinic was a very high success rate when people opted to use the raw Chinese herbs. The less processed western herbal tinctures also worked well, but there was still something missing. For me, I always wondered if the processing of a herb, which meant the more interference with it, decreased the effectiveness due to not respecting the plant spirit.

In both Western and Chinese Medicine we look at the individual as a whole. Emotions, environment, diet – everything is taken into consideration when looking at an imbalance and the cause. But when it comes to prescribing herbs, we look at the physical action on the body, and not what a herb can do with the emotional or spiritual body. In Western Herbal Medicine, we could also use flower essences to address emotional or behavioural issues.

A person's lifestyle, behaviours or emotional status may be the major factor contributing to or creating their illness and this needs to be addressed. We learn at university how these factors have a big impact on the body, but we don't address the many ways to change them. Some issues are obvious, and others are multi-layered. Sometimes it is not our place to delve into matters that we are not trained in, so why then are we not trained in these matters more fully?

There are subjects that a university will not touch on generally because they will never get it passed through the appropriate channels. This is where Plant Spirit Medicine falls. I doubt in my lifetime anyone will be able to go to uni to learn about shamanic principles, like that of soul loss and journeying to meet plant spirits. This is where our disconnect lies in our healing training. Obviously, we are able to refer people on to psychologists and counsellors, and these modalities can also help greatly, but there is still the spiritual healing side of things that is so grossly left untouched and so needed at this time. This is why there has been such growth in the spiritual industry – people are searching for their own answers and healing.

Soul loss is an important area in shamanism. When we experience trauma, sometimes it can be too much for the soul or spirit to handle. The soul is then said to fragment, and these fragments can remain trapped in that time and experience, too afraid to move forward. Our soul can fragment many times over our lifetimes and also in previous lives as well. This causes a feeling of being not quite ourselves and can manifest as illnesses that won't budge or patterns that keep playing out in our lives and we can't understand why. This is where we would call on a shaman to journey for us to find our missing soul pieces, ask them to come back and let them know it is now safe for them to return. I have experienced profound changes within myself after completing these exercises.

Celtic shamanism

There are many forms of shamanism around the world and each have their own deities and totem animals, but all have common traits that link them. Shamanism is not a religion; it is a spiritual practice. It can be practised alongside any religion or not encompass religion at all. It is not about worship; it's about respect for nature and every living creature on earth. It's about becoming one with nature's cycles and learning that we are a part of everything. Spirit resides in every living creature on this planet, and shamans believe we can communicate with all living beings because we are all created by spirit, and we are spirit. People may view shamans as having a special ability – however, my belief is that anyone is capable of this. It's just that, as a species, we have forgotten how to do it.

Why have I chosen Celtic shamanism? Being of Scottish descent, perhaps that's why I was drawn to it – ancestrally, it is in my blood. I cannot describe it, but I have always felt drawn to my heritage. As I looked into Celtic shamanism more and more, it made so much sense to me. I really resonated with the teachings.

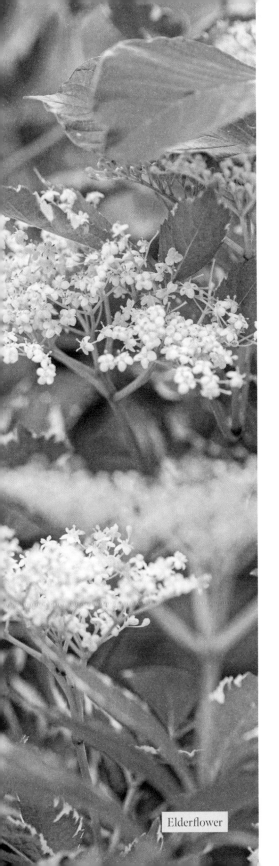

Elderflower

The Celts are recognised as being from Ireland, Scotland, England and Wales; however, many Celts came from all over Europe and incorporated their own practices with those of the indigenous people of the United Kingdom. The Celts themselves actually never used the word 'shamanism'. They called such people 'walkers between the worlds'. They were seen as being interpreters of the spirit realms. In other countries, shamans are described as 'having one foot in both worlds', which again indicates their ability to communicate with other realms. A natural gift for many Celts, second sight (da shealladh) enabled a person to have visions, strong intuition and divinatory abilities, and was another way they could communicate with other-world beings.

Western society has lost a significant portion of the knowledge our ancestors once had, knowledge that allowed our ancestors to understand the workings of nature and our part in it. They knew they were not separate from the world around them but were part of it. They worked in harmony, and if only there had not been such a disruption in their practices I can only imagine where we would be now. This knowledge is still practised in many indigenous cultures around the world. Regardless of which continent they are from, the indigenes have many common practices, but most importantly they have respect for all of nature and creation both big and small.

As torrid as our history is, with the desecration of certain cultures and things such as the witch trials, there is nothing we can do to change what has been done. The only thing we can do is realise we are in a modern society in which times and views are radically changing, and it is now a safe time to bring back the old ways and respect all cultures and life on this earth. In saying that, we do not need to be constrained in exactly how these old ways were practised; it's about taking the knowledge we do have and creating a new vision for the modern world.

I feel there are no longer enough healers on this earth to make the difference that is needed

I feel there are no longer enough healers on this earth to make the difference that is needed. It is time for the healers to become teachers and empower others to take their spiritual growth into their own hands, to help them navigate and understand the workings of nature so they can use their knowledge to help themselves and teach their children. This needs to happen on a mass scale to bring the balance back to earth before there is no turning back. People are beginning to understand the importance of this, and are becoming more awake and aware.

Each day I feel more and more grateful for my connection to everything, for my understanding of the world. You don't need to be a shaman to practise Plant Spirit Medicine; just know that, whatever way you choose to work with the plant spirits, respect, love and authenticity are the keys. Regardless of whether you feel or see anything when working with them, please know you are making connections purely through your intentions, respect and sincerity.

Here also is where Plant Spirit Medicine comes in. I like to think of it as 'Spirit' Medicine. This medicine allows us to step back and allow the plant spirit to help the human spirit. It can help us see patterns and behaviours we are acting out that are having a detrimental effect on our lives. They can help us to look at things differently, so we become more in alignment with our higher selves.

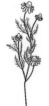

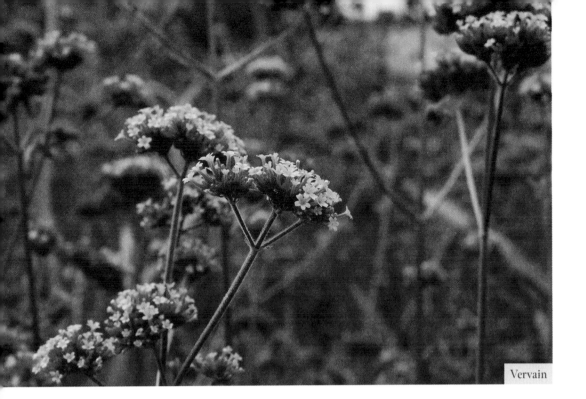

My vervain experience

Vervain is traditionally known for its ability to clear through obstacles and for being the herb of love. I have worked with the vervain plant spirit and am in awe of what it showed me. It helped me break free of the issues holding me back from finding true love.

> *When I journeyed to meet the plant spirit, I couldn't make contact for some reason. So I bought the raw herb and under ritual made a small elixir with the vervain mixed into wine. During the ritual, I literally felt the vervain plant spirit with me and imbue into the mix as I was stirring it. I had never felt this before, so I was pretty excited. But trust me, the taste is awful as vervain is very astringent/bitter, so don't waste too much wine if you ever do it!*

In the space of a few months, I had old boyfriends contact me out of the blue – some I hadn't seen in close to 30 years! They all told me the same thing: that they were sorry they had let me go and that it wasn't me, it was them, or they found it so hard leaving but knew they had to pursue their careers etc. It allowed me to see that not every break-up was because of me, like I had thought. I had such low self-esteem, I had woven into my story that I wasn't good enough and that's why people left me. I hadn't seen the situation for what it was, and that there were other factors that contributed to the break-ups. This insight allowed me to let go of a lot of hurt and see my situation from another angle. Letting go of all that energy tied up in the hurt gave me room to love myself and also to allow love in. Not only was my self-esteem boosted, I felt empowered and ready for love, and realised the partner I am now with was in front of my eyes all along. You see, you attract what you are. I had not been attracted to him at that time, because he was not holding on to the same baggage that I was. He did not have the low self-esteem that I had. We were not a match at that time, but when I let go of my baggage I became in vibrational alignment with him. End of story.

The other lesson I learned from this experience was that there is only so much you can learn from journeying to meet a plant spirit. Sometimes it needs to be experienced first hand, so vervain is one of my go-to herbs when needing to work through areas of love, self-love and self-esteem.

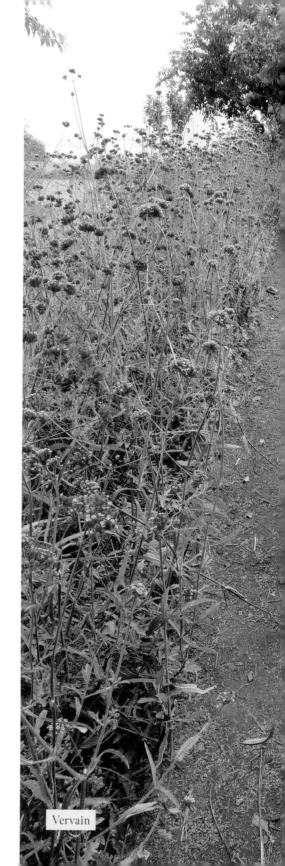

Vervain

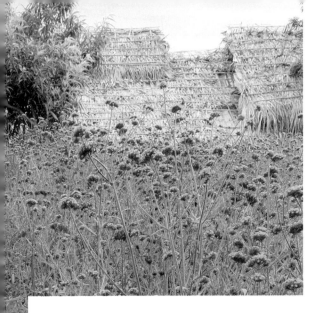

There are many aspects to making herbal preparations that you must be aware of

Plant Spirit Medicine in essence teaches us how to see ourselves. It can show us what we need to let go of to heal our traumas so we can become the person we are meant to be. The plants are so willing to help us if we ask them. They know that as we heal, we evolve – and evolve we must!

This book is on Plant Spirit Medicine making. In these pages, I wish to show you how the herbalist becomes the conduit or the bridge for the plant spirit to imbue into the herbal products.

There are many aspects to making herbal preparations that you must be aware of. Especially the legal implications. It is important to thoroughly understand what you are making as you must harm no one. You must keep in mind at all times that, even though we are working with the plant spirits, the physical properties of the herbs/plants in our products also have actions on the physical body. We don't want to be making something toxic that the client ingests, for example, or making a cream that can cause skin reactions. Knowing how to create safely and abide by your governing laws should be your utmost priority while creating. I don't want to deter you from making them or instil fear into you, I just see too many people not researching properly and not adhering to the laws, and so I wish to ensure that you start off with the right way of doing things from the get-go. Another thing I will do is flip between the spiritual and physical properties of some of the herbs/plants because you can't really separate the two. We are using the physical plant in most cases, so there will always be an effect of some kind to the physical body, and this always needs to be kept in mind for the safety of you and/or your client.

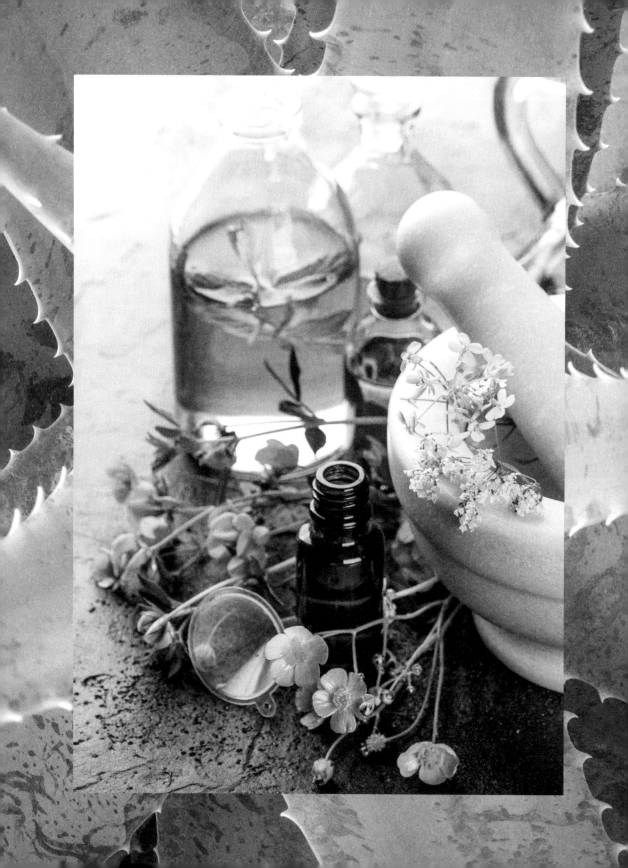

CHAPTER 2

Cycles and seasons

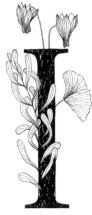

I f we want to attune ourselves better to nature, we must attune ourselves to its cycles and seasons. Why should we attune ourselves to nature to make Plant Spirit Medicine? Because we are tuning into Source energy. This Source energy manifests itself through nature. We are part of this energy – therefore, we are also part of nature. For us to work closely with the plant spirits of nature, we must align ourselves with that which we have created a perceived separation from. This is an important key to working with this medicine. We must get out into nature. We must spend time there. Whenever I travel, I always manage to find at least a small park or a beautiful tree to sit under. You don't have to have money or a car to travel to find somewhere – there should be no excuses. Nature is everywhere – even if you get yourself a pot plant or turn a city balcony into a plant oasis. Take cuttings from people's plants if you can't afford your own. There is always a way to get yourself closer to nature. Find it. Once you discover this connection, your world will never be the same. It's like coming home, and you never want to be separated from it again.

When I moved to Tamborine Mountain, I went through a very tumultuous time in my life. I didn't have any money to do anything, so I started going for bushwalks on the mountain. I was literally terrified to walk by myself, so I would pick up a big stick to walk with, and I would jump at the slightest sound. I did the same walk about three times a week, about three kilometres, and halfway I would sit at the waterfall and do a little meditation or just soak up the sounds of the water and watch the birds in the trees. At the time, I was also learning about Celtic shamanism, so I started trying to connect to the forest each time I went. As I was walking in, I would say hello and I would picture my energy field expanding as I walked, as if it was blending with the forest energy. I would also picture my animal spirit guides walking in front of me and behind me to check the path. I would ask them to warn me of any potential dangers. Over time, every time I did the same walk, I felt a part of the forest. I no longer felt afraid, and I began to know all the sounds, all the birds, all the trees and all the cycles the forest would go through. I would see trees being eaten from the inside by termites that eventually would fall down and clear a path through the forest, only to then become forest floor food and nutrients for the soil and a foundation for the fungus and moss to grow on. In time I felt welcomed, and the forest became my magical home away from home.

> I discovered that I could go to the forest with specific questions and walk out with solutions

The other thing I noticed was that when I walked in with a mind full of clutter and questions, I would walk out calm and with answers. I discovered that I could go to the forest with specific questions and walk out with solutions without having to truly work it out in my head. I realised I was tapping into something normally overlooked. I noticed how people would walk into the forest and talk the entire time they were there. I love to walk in total silence. This not only allows you to be alone with your thoughts, but to pick up on everything that is happening around you and for you to receive guidance from the plant spirits all around you.

Many indigenous tribes claim that plants have a particular song or vibration specific to each plant, that this is how they can find it, hear it and know it. Maybe next time you are in the garden or go on a bushwalk, walk silently and see if any tunes or notes come to you.

When we align ourselves with nature, we get in the flow of the cycles and seasons. When it is winter, we should be slowing down, conserving energy and eating more dense nourishing foods to replenish our bodies. This is a great time to relax more and

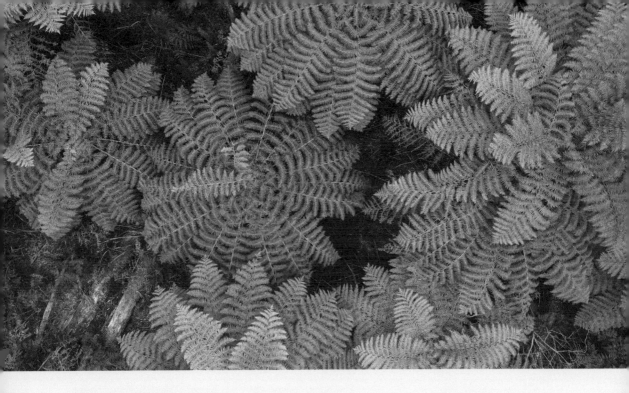

maybe cultivate our ideas for the coming spring. Spring comes and we find ourselves wanting to spring clean and start new projects, just like the gardens that are now coming to life and taking off. Summer is a high-energy period and one when we can easily overdo things. Autumn starts to slow us down a bit and this is a good time to start letting things go, just as the trees drop their leaves.

We also have the cycles of the moon, which we know play an important role in gardening. The energy of a plant builds towards the full moon and then wanes heading to the new moon. Knowing these cycles and being aware of the ebb and flow can give you an indication of the best times to be picking your plant for your medicine making. Do you want the strong vibrant energy of it, or do you need the calming, withdrawing part of it? Do you want to brew your medicine over a full moon cycle or just one night on the full moon?

If we are using the root, for instance, we might want to harvest it in winter when the energy of the plant is stored mainly in the root. Or we might want to make a St John's wort–infused oil. You actually need to use the flowering tops to create this oil, which turns it a beautiful red. So if you intend to grow the herb and harvest the flowers, you will need to learn at what point it will flower. The more you get to know the growth cycle of a plant, the closer you will become to it.

Doctrine of signatures

In my Western Herbal Medicine degree, I learned this amazing thing called the doctrine of signatures. This doctrine states that herbs/plants that resemble particular parts of the body can be used to treat ailments of those body parts, and that the plant's location, habits, colour and form give clues as to how and when it can be used. Thus, healers have come to understand the uses of herbs simply by observing the plant's conditions, locality and characteristics: its colour, where it grew, how animals used it, when it flowers etc.

Let's look at aloe vera as an example, which we know is great for sunburn. Its doctrine of signature shows that it loves the sun and is full of moisture inside. Its main action is to give moisture back to your skin after exposure to the sun.

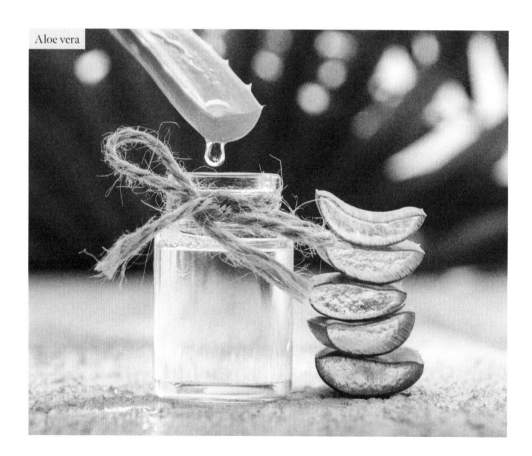

Aloe vera

Another strong signature is that of the ginkgo tree, the leaves of which demonstrate what it's best used for. The leaves are very similar in shape to the two lobes of the brain, the eye with its optic nerve, the kidneys and the lungs. It comes as no surprise that it helps to supply blood and oxygen to all of those body parts.

In Chinese medicine, flowers that grow up and open generally work on releasing pathogens from the upper body, such as in the eyes and sinuses. Even the humble walnut, the nut of which looks like a brain, has beneficial effects on the brain. Nature really is amazing.

The doctrine may relate to where it grows and how it grows. Does it grow within the rocks or in swampy soil? Some doctrines can be seen by the colour of the plant, whether it requires lots of water or if it grows in the desert. Some doctrines are hard to tell and some you might not find at all. The more you observe and research, the more you will find.

Always take note of the plants that grow where you live. Plants grow where they are needed. Sometimes you might move to somewhere and something starts to pop up that used to live where you moved from. This might be an indication that this is a Plant Spirit Medicine that you need, especially if you have noticed it and thought it unusual.

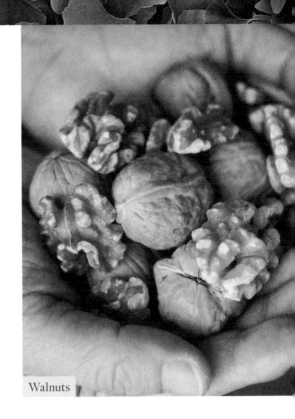

Walnuts

Even the humble walnut, the nut of which looks like a brain, has beneficial effects on the brain

Tree of Life exercise

Whenever I do any form of energy or spiritual work, I ground myself first. This process alone performed every day is enough to spark a massive shift in your life. I practised it every day for three months, and it was literally life changing, so don't underestimate the significance of grounding and protecting your energy. It's a good idea to do this before you start any spiritual exercise.

I do this exercise standing, to feel as much like a tree as possible. You may have your own way of doing it, so do whatever feels comfortable for you. The Tree of Life exercise is an extremely valuable part of any spiritual undertaking, creating your connection to the earth and to the energies above. You should draw your energy from it just as the tree draws its energy through its roots and leaves.

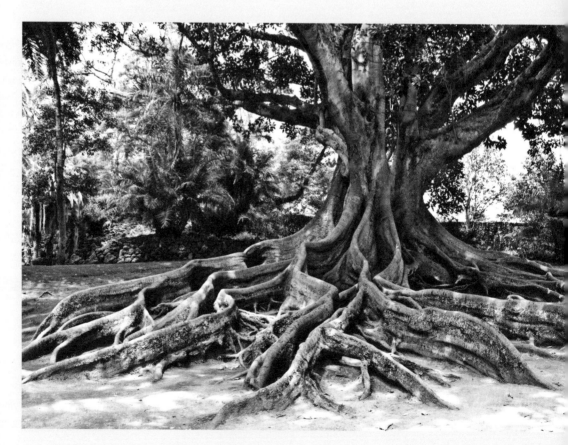

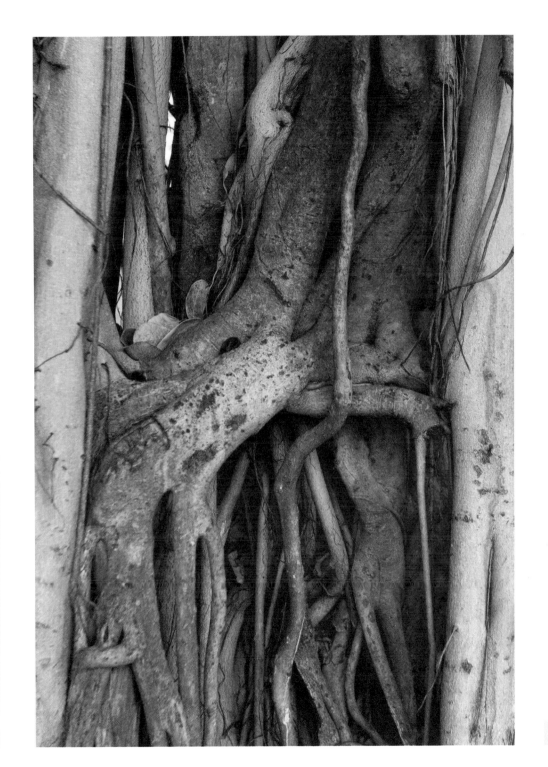

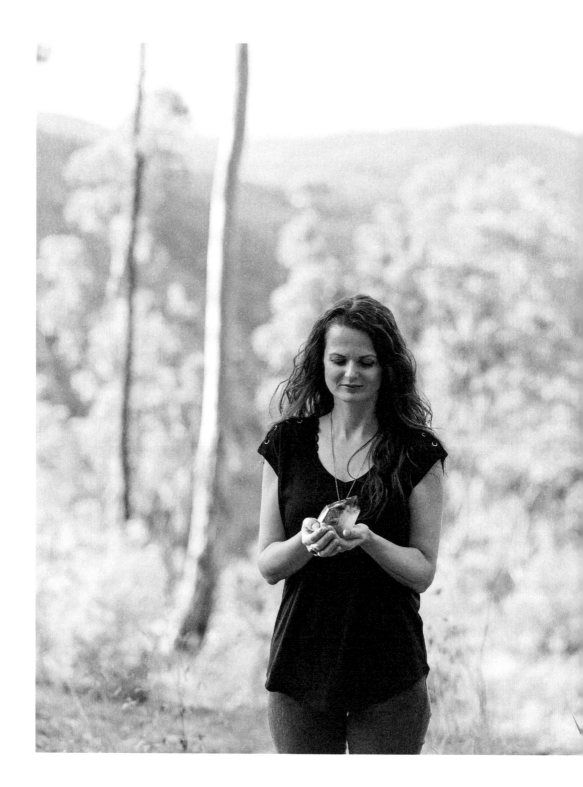

To ground and connect:

- **Stand comfortably with your feet shoulder-width apart and unlock your knees.** You can also do this lying down or sitting up in a seat. Find your centre and breathe out all your tension.

- **If you are standing, rock back and forth on your feet a little to find a good position,** so that your balance becomes distributed evenly over your feet, and make sure you unlock your knees. Let them bend a little. You will feel any areas of tension that you need to let go of.

- **Close your eyes and take a few deep breaths to relax and focus.** Picture roots growing out of your feet and tailbone and into the earth. Send the roots down through the earth. See them pushing through all the layers of the earth.

- **Picture a big white ball of energy in the centre of the earth.** Connect your roots to the ball of light. Picture the light from this ball moving up through your roots, like a tree drawing up water and nutrients from the soil. Draw this light up through the soles of your feet and tailbone. Draw the light up through your body to your heart. It may be easier to draw the energy up on every in-breath to create a good rhythm.

- **See the light go down to your fingertips and back to your heart.** See the light go up through the centre of your head. See it extending out through branches sprouting from your head, shoulders and arms. Lift your arms to also draw the power up and to feel and become the tree. Send the energy out through the ends of the branches and out through the leaves into the sky. Watch it extend up through the layers of the atmosphere into space, and reach up to touch the sun or moon (depending on the time of day) or perhaps a star.

- **Feel the sun, moon or star light on your face** as you draw down its white light through your head, and trace the way back that the earth light came through you. Down through your head, to your heart, to your fingertips and back to your heart, down through your body, out through your feet and through the roots, and connect with the ball of white light in the centre of the earth.

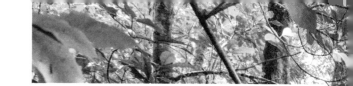

Now that you have connected like the Tree of Life, it is important to shield yourself. This will help deflect any negative energies but will also contain the energy you now have flowing through you.

Picture a big white or gold bubble in front of you that you step into, or maybe a shield pops up all around you. Go with whatever feels right for you. Fill your shield full of white light and know you are protected. Now you can proceed with your exercise/ritual.

Attuning with nature exercise

For this exercise, we are going to learn to connect to nature. You can do the exercise on a special walk, in a park, your backyard or even next to your pot plant. Outdoors is best, and when starting out try to be somewhere as quiet as possible. Make sure you won't be disturbed, and either switch your phone off or into airplane mode.

Find a nice place to sit with nature. Sit in front of a plant that you are drawn to, a patch of grass that looks inviting, or if you are on a walk find somewhere you are not going to be disturbed. Sit in a comfortable position so there is nothing to distract you. Calm yourself by taking long, slow breaths. Every time you exhale, feel more tension drain out of your body. In your head or out loud if you prefer, say to your plant, tree or forest: 'Hello. I ask to make contact with you. Please show me or guide me how to communicate with you,' then push your energy field out from your body. Feel it expand, then feel it expand more and more until your energy field stretches out and co-mingles with all your surroundings. Sit in this moment and focus on the silence, the wind in the trees, the birds chirping. Shift any thoughts that come into your head out of the way and keep returning to just 'being' and feeling the co-mingling of your energy fields. Do you hear any song or notes?

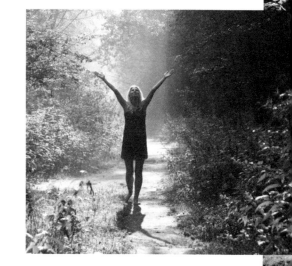

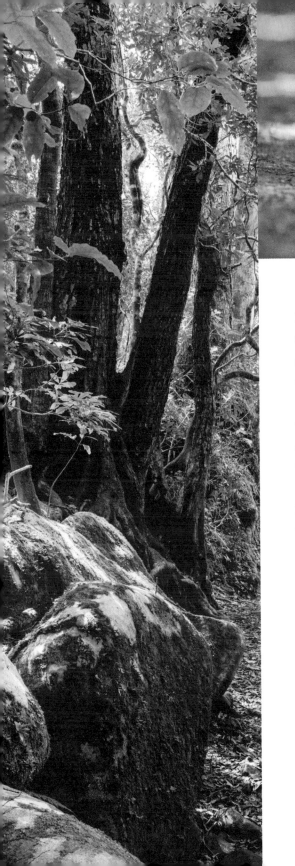

Do you see or hear any messages being given to you from the plant? Maybe you can feel something. Stay here for a few minutes and take it in. Don't analyse, just let it flow.

Once you feel it is time to come back, thank the plant, tree or forest for their contact, pull in your energy field and feel yourself back in your body.

This can be repeated as many times as you like. It's also a great exercise to do before you walk into a forest or anywhere in nature. You can do this with your eyes open and walking. When you leave the forest, say thank you and draw your energy field in before leaving. You might also want to leave an offering of gratitude. If you don't have anything with you, just sending your love and gratitude is enough. You could pour a little water at the base of your plant to say thank you. Please don't leave gifts that are not biodegradable.

Make this a common practice in your life. It's quick and easy, and it has some really remarkable benefits.

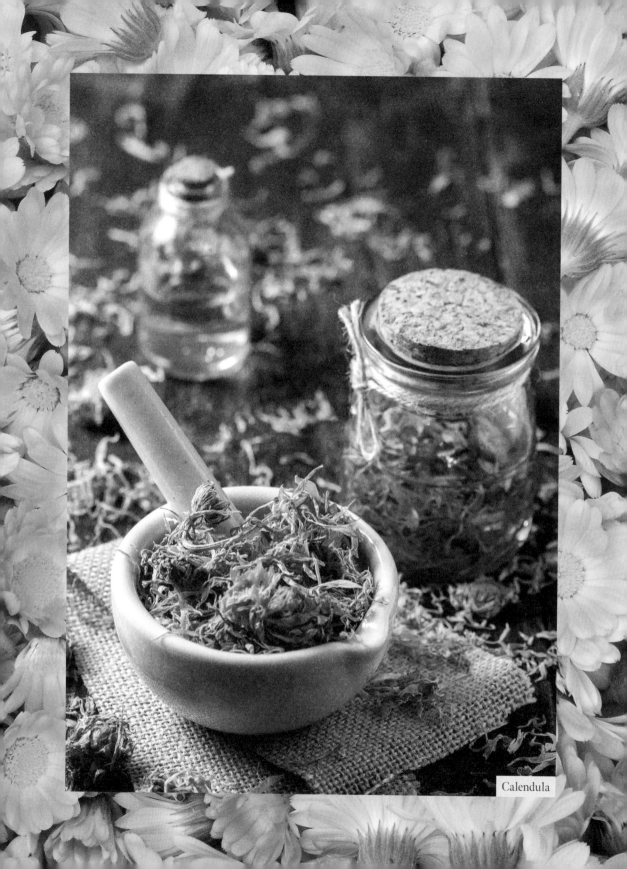

Calendula

CHAPTER 3

Laws, plant identification and safety

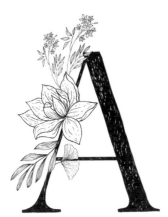

ll plant medicine should be treated with the utmost respect and safety. It is also important to understand modern-day government restrictions that need to be adhered to. You should research your herbs thoroughly to ensure you understand them well enough to avoid using something toxic to the skin or body, or something endangered or illegal. You also need to be able to identify your plant, know what research is needed and what labelling requirements you need for your products.

Keep in mind we are focusing on Plant Spirit Medicine making, so many of the rules don't apply because essentially you are not making any physical therapeutic claims; however, we must keep in mind that they very well may have a physiological effect, so we need to know exactly what we are making. We always have to take both into consideration. With anything we apply to the body, ingest or even spray into the air that we will breathe in, it's imperative to be safe and mindful about what we are doing, what we are using and where it will be applied. Please also be mindful of pets that may also breathe in what is sprayed or burnt in the air.

Government restrictions

It is extremely important to adhere to the laws in your country. The use of the word 'medicine' may get you into trouble. Even though I am a registered herbalist within Australia, I am not allowed to make any claims about any of my products. I cannot say you can use my salve for physical conditions like eczema, for example, even though it very well may work for that condition. I'm not even allowed to have testimonials stating that my products worked for a specific condition. You can understand how extremely difficult it is to market yourself and your products if you can't actually say what you can treat and what your products are made for. Beware using the word 'treat' as well, as this implies a therapeutic claim. Even saying that the herbs in your creation are traditionally used for ... may not be allowed, as it insinuates that your product does what it traditionally says it does. Unfortunately, there are many people who either don't know the rules around therapeutic claims or have decided not to worry about it, out there promoting all their healing products and themselves, while I have to sit back and hold my tongue.

I understand why these laws are in place. It's easy to read some information on what a herb does, then put it in a formulation and think your product will work for you in this way. It certainly may, but there are also a lot of factors with plants that you need to be aware of, and when you have studied and researched properly you understand this.

There are so many factors with herbs and plants you need to take into consideration when making products. Therapeutic products need to have specific levels of active constituents in order for them to be effective. The levels of these constituents will vary depending on where the plant is grown in terms of country and locality, it's growing conditions, harvesting time and methods including proper storage. You might buy dried calendula that has been stored for too long, picked too early, grown in poor soil and harvested at the wrong time. These flowers will not give you a good-quality calendula oil if you infuse them. You then make a product from this oil stating that it is good for eczema, and people unwittingly buy your product because you have claimed it works – and it's only then they find it really doesn't.

You might also be making a calendula oil infusion that is too weak, where the active constituents have not been extracted effectively because you were unaware calendula needs 90% alcohol for effective extraction, and you have placed it in oil only. Again, this means that your end product won't be as effective as you claim it to be. Any benefit the customer might be getting from the product would be from the oil they are rubbing into their skin and not necessarily the calendula.

When making home-made herbal products it is impossible to determine the levels of your active constituents; it is impossible to test your products consistency to prove every tin or jar of your product has the same outcome. This is why in Australia, for example, products are contract manufactured on a large scale within a good manufacturing practice (GMP) facility. These facilities have extensive protocols in place to ensure your product is made to strict guidelines and that every product is of the highest standard. When this is achieved, you can then apply to the Therapeutic

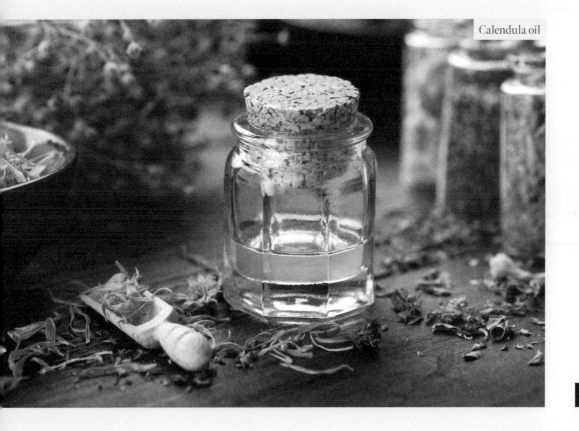

Calendula oil

Goods Administration (TGA) to list your product as a therapeutic product and pay a fee. You also need to have all the supporting documentation and research to back up your claims, which can be a lengthy procedure. You then receive a number that needs to be placed on your product, and from there you are able to make your claims.

Many other countries have even more strict guidelines where, even if you are just making products from home, you have to have them tested for safety, which can cost thousands of dollars.

As a herbalist within Australia, I am allowed to make therapeutic products for my clients, however, I am only allowed to make them up per client. I am certainly not allowed to make up batches and sell them individually, claiming what they can be used for.

My point here is: *do not make any therapeutic claims* about your products if you are not allowed to in your country.

So what can you claim on your products?

Because we are working with Plant *Spirit* Medicine, we are working with emotional and spiritual conditions. Therefore, you shouldn't need to make any physical claims. However, you will need to know any cautions that people should be aware of – for example, for pregnant women etc. If you are using a herb that is a muscle relaxant or can stimulate the uterus if applied to the belly, you need to add the warning to your label. If you use St John's wort in a product to go on the skin, sometimes this can create photosensitivity in some people, and you must add this in your information somewhere.

You cannot control how people use your product, and people will be creative in how they use it; they may overdo it because they think it's natural, so it can't harm them. Do not underestimate the power of herbs – overusing anything can have harmful effects. We will get to labelling in more detail later – but keep these things in mind.

Hopefully, you are not too alarmed by all of this. I was, for a long time, which caused a big roadblock for me, and this is why I started off with basic skincare. You can use words like moisturising or hydrating for your skin and other terminology for your products, or you can just be creative and come up with something that describes how you might feel when you use the product – for example: 'Enjoy the luxurious feeling of pampering your skin with the beautiful hydrating qualities of …'

Here is an example of the Plant Spirit Medicine terminology I use for my mugwort balm:

> *Mugwort is traditionally known for its visionary actions. It is said to help aid prophecies and dreamwork, strengthen psychic powers and astral projection. [I have used the words 'traditionally known' here, but keep in mind it is not used to describe a therapeutic action.]*

CAUTION: *if you have sensitive skin, do a skin test first as mugwort is high in volatile oils. Care should be taken or avoided if you are pregnant, as mugwort is a muscle relaxant. In saying that, a small amount on your body or tools is obviously fine, and you will still be able to work with the plant spirit. Just don't go rubbing it all over your belly if you are pregnant.*

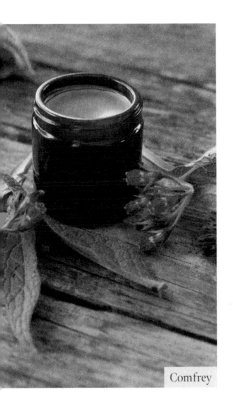

Comfrey

Banned herbs

In Australia there is a list of scheduled herbs, which means they generally have restrictions on them due to their potential toxicities or vulnerability due to over-harvesting. Research your herbs to ensure you are not using anything that is actually illegal to use in your country, even if you think it is safe. Comfrey, at the time of writing this book, is a scheduled herb in Australia although it has been used widely for centuries. There are guidelines to adhere to when using it, so it hasn't been completely taken from us, but it is a great example of why we need to research. It is allowed to be used in topical applications, but not internal. The scheduled herbs list can change from time to time, so always keep checking back. Check your country's legislation regarding scheduled herbs on the relevant government website.

Plant identification

This can be another tricky topic. Sometimes we are drawn to a plant and have no idea what it is, and even if we do there may not be any information on how it can be applied. This is where it is imperative to communicate with your plant to discover how it needs to be used. If you are new to Plant Spirit Medicine and/or herbalism, please start with something that you know is safe. I will give you a list of safe and well-known herbs to get you started later.

You don't even need the physical plant to receive its healing, because it is the spirit of the plant that works on the emotional and spiritual aspects of oneself. So, if in doubt, just ask the plant spirit for its healing.

Knowing the botanical/Latin name is best as this generally remains consistent around the world. This is also their scientific name – for example, rosemary is known as *Rosmarinus officinalis* and lavender is known is *Lavandula angustifolia*. There may be many species of the one plant depending on what type. For example, there is French lavender, which is *L. stoechas*, and then English lavender, which is *L. angustifolia.* If in doubt buy the seeds and grow your own, or purchase from a reputable herb nursery.

There are many resources you can use to identify a plant. There are phone apps where you can take a photo and it will tell you. There

> If in doubt buy the seeds and grow your own, or purchase from a reputable herb nursery

are forums. You could take a photo and take it to your local nursery, herb or plant club. You could visit your local library or join up online, join a gardening club or purchase a herbal pharmacopoeia. I love to go to the local book fests and pick up herb books for a couple of dollars. I also like to buy seeds from a reputable seller and grow them myself. What better way to get to know a plant than growing it yourself, nurturing it, learning what it needs and then making your own medicine from it? This way you can establish a lasting relationship with the plant while creating an environmentally friendly and sustainable product.

Even if you think you know what a plant is, it's a good idea to look it up. Let's take the common dandelion for example: *Taraxacum officinale*. Most of us have grown up making wishes blowing dandelion seeds into the wind. Did you know there is a strikingly similar plant that many mistake for true dandelion? This is what it looks like:

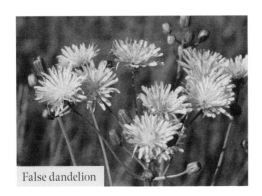
False dandelion

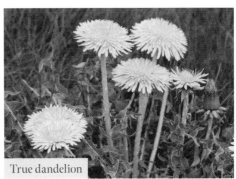
True dandelion

This is called by many names: false dandelion, catsear, flatweed and its scientific name, *Hypochaeris radicata*. See how close it resembles true dandelion?

Can you spot the differences?

Although they look very similar, the easiest way to distinguish between the two is a true dandelion flower will have one hollow stem per flower, and they are generally bigger. False dandelion will have a branched stem with more than one flower, and the stem is solid. The leaves are similar also, but dandelion leaves come to a pointed tip and false dandelions are rounded, with the leaves lying more flat to the ground. In noticing the differences between these two plants, you can see why it is imperative to get your plant identification correct. Thankfully, in this case, both plants are ok to consume, but this is not always so.

Which part of the plant do you use?

Keep in mind again that we are working with the plant spirit and not making therapeutic products, although you may be doing both. Either way, you need to research your specific herb/plant. Sometimes only the flowers are used. Other times it may be the leaves or the roots. There are way too many plants to go through in detail here, so it's best left to you to research your own plant. The plant spirit may guide you to use something that isn't normally used, and this is still ok. It means the plant spirit will be with you and the product, but don't expect to sell or use it as the therapeutic version.

Wildcrafting vs cultivation

Work responsible and be environmentally friendly. What we create must have little to no impact on the earth. There is a big debate on wildcrafting vs cultivation. There are pros and cons to both. Unfortunately, there are

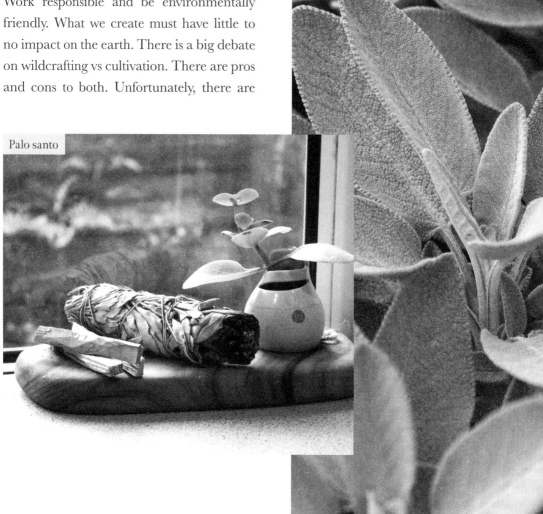

Palo santo

greedy people in the world and wildcrafting to them equates to free herbs and they take more than is required, leaving none for anyone else and depleting a plant to the point of extinction in some cases. This is why cultivation is sometimes needed, so we don't deplete the natural environment. It's important to fully know your botany when wildcrafting so you know exactly what you are picking. There have been many cases of the wrong plant being used as it looked similar to the correct plant.

Herbs like white sage and wood like palo santo are amazing plants used for smudge. However, since being introduced to the Western world, both are now on the brink of exhaustion and/or becoming endangered. Over-harvesting, unethical and unsustainable practices are taking place, and if we are to protect them we must make an educated decision when buying them. On one hand we don't want to put the reputable sellers out of business who work in a sustainable manner, but we do wish to deter the unethical dealers. We also need to take into consideration that these are sacred plants to their native people, who have established a relationship with them. We must respect these plants, and if they wish to work with us they will make themselves known. I now grow my own white sage.

… if we are to protect them we must make an educated decision when buying them

We also must take into consideration the use of sprayed chemicals on plants or chemicals from run-off. You might think twice about collecting herbs from the roadside as they may have been sprayed by the council or polluted by the volume of car exhausts driving by them each day. Consider the run-off from neighbouring properties, which could be air-born particles or from a direct water source. ***Please do not use contaminated products.***

There are many options we can use to substitute for both of these plants in our practice, and I highly suggest growing plants to use yourself as smudge or find something local to your area. This again will help you make a strong connection with the plant spirits. There is more on making your own smudge sticks in Chapter 7.

Safe herbal list

How do we select which plant/s we want to make our medicine from? This will depend on where you live. You might have herbs growing in your garden that you are familiar with already. It's always best to start out with something you know is safe and you can find a lot of information on. For example:

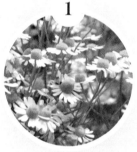

1

German chamomile

Matricaria recutita

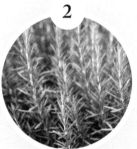

2

Rosemary

Rosmarinus officinalis

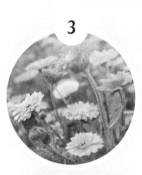

3

Calendula

Calendula officinalis

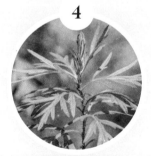

4

Mugwort

Artemisia vulgaris

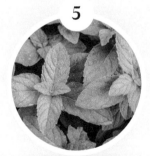

5

Peppermint

Mentha piperita

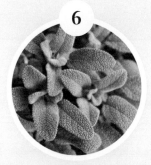

Sage

Salvia miltiorrhiza

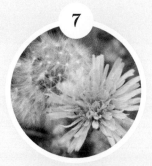

Dandelion

Taraxacum officinale

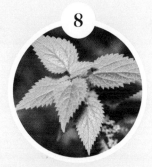

Nettle

Urtica dioica

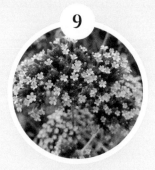

Vervain

Verbena officinalis

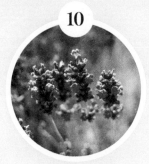

Lavender

Lavandula angustifolia

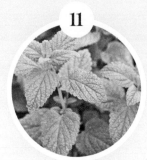

Lemon balm

Melissa officinalis

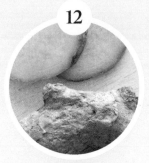

Ginger

Zingiber officinale

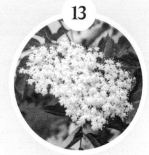

Elderflower

Sambucus nigra

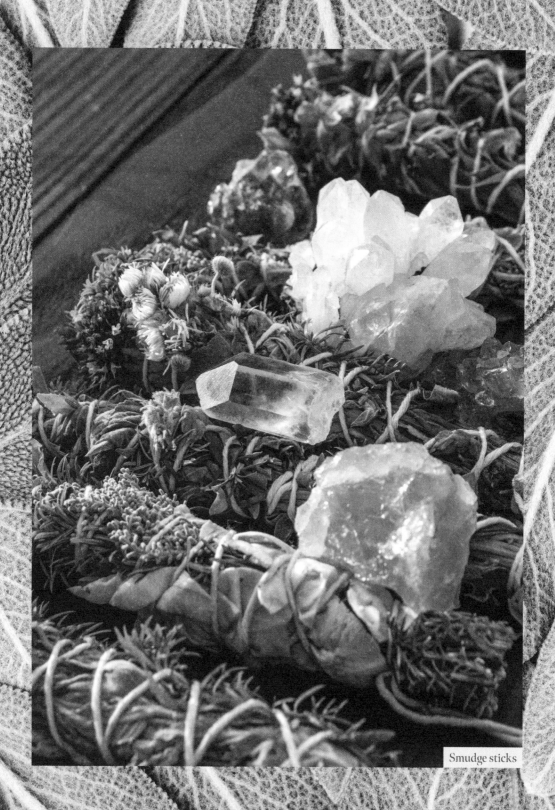

Smudge sticks

CHAPTER 4

Plant connections and ritual

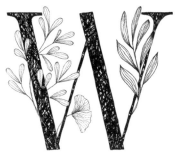

When making Plant Spirit Medicine, we work in ritual and with the plant spirit throughout the whole process. They are present and will guide you. It is also important for you to actually participate in the activities, as you need to connect to the plant to understand them and for them to want to work with you. It's easy to become complacent or rush things once you've made them a few times. You can certainly speed up the process once you know what you are doing, but when starting out it is best to take your time until you feel what is going on. The most important thing to remember is:

> *Be sure to ask the plant for its healing and wisdom and be respectful at all times. Intent is key.*

Don't go ripping plants up or just jumping into creating and then asking later. You must be mindful and respectful throughout the whole process, even down to discarding waste into your garden and not just throwing it in your rubbish bin. Treat everything as sacred and respect it.

Don't feel that you have to be a spiritual guru in order to make a connection to a plant either. It's hard to know what to expect when you've never done it. Keep in mind plants have a different way of communicating than we do, and that is what we need to focus on. When we think of communication, we think of the spoken word. Plants don't generally communicate this way, and it takes practice to understand the way in which they do communicate. For instance, you might be really drawn to a plant. This could be its way of communicating with you and you are responding. When I do shamanic journeying I see the plant or plant spirit, and it communicates through images. Here's an example from when I performed a journey to meet the blackberry plant spirit:

As I journeyed to the middle world (one of the three worlds in shamanism), I found myself in a beautiful open meadow. The weather was overcast. I realised I was in England out the back of an old house, with a blackberry bush surrounding the perimeter. I kept seeing a black being with no face or features, just literally a shape. I moved closer to the big patch of blackberry. The shape pulled me inside the tangle of bushes, and in there I understood how protective blackberry is with masses of it all around me, and yet even though there were so many bushes it didn't feel constricting. The sun shone through the thicket and inside the air was fresh. It felt safe. There was a sense of refuge there and a means to be able to travel within it safely. The plant spirit took ahold of both my hands and I felt him enter me. Looking out of my eyes, he was trying to show me to look out of my third eye. I felt goodwill and love and then he departed, and I came back.

I am a visual person, so spirit communicates with me this way. What I took from this journey was that the blackberry is a protective plant – a plant I could call on when I needed to find safety or sanctuary. From that space I could also feel safe while travelling, whether physically or spiritually speaking.

You need to find your way of communicating. It may be visual; it could be through feeling, knowing, smelling, hearing; or it could be like the vervain plant medicine I encountered, where I had to physically experience it. The point is, you need to ask

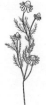

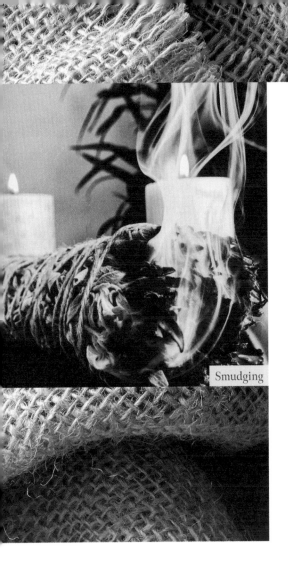

Smudging

... when I
speak my truth
and lay it out
there it is well
received most
of the time

the plant spirit if it can show you. Ask it for its healing, wisdom and guidance.

I'm also totally aware in this day and age that Plant Spirit Medicine is looked down upon and seen as spiritual mumbo jumbo. I find myself at times filtering what I say to certain people as I know they don't believe in what I do. I don't judge them for not believing in this medicine; I probably wouldn't have believed it when I was younger. For me, I understand that everyone is on their own path, and we all have different beliefs. If you wish to step into this area of work and are hesitant about putting yourself out there, please don't feel that you have to. You can still make beautiful products. As long as you know you have worked respectfully with the plant to create your product, you will draw to you the people who resonate with it whether they understand it or not. I have found, though, that when I speak my truth and lay it out there it is well received most of the time. There will always be someone who doesn't believe, so don't take it personally. Do what feels right for you.

The ritual of Plant Spirit Medicine making

The ritual of working with the plant spirit is the most important step in medicine making. We need to be working with the plant at all stages where possible. You can make this as elaborate or simple as you like; your intent

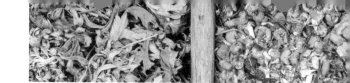

and focus is always key here. I find the more effort I put in with creating space, like putting on my special jewellery, lighting a candle, using specific tools etc., the more it helps me create the focus and atmosphere I need to connect more wholly.

If the word ritual feels foreign to you, please find what sits right with you. A ritual can be anything from having a cup of tea each morning, allowing you to relax and start your day.

A ritual should be a practice that shifts you out of everyday reality and allows you to be present to focus on your intent.

I want to make it clear that no matter what faith, religion or spiritual practice you follow, the energy is one and the same. The tools and the rituals we use are created by us to help connect to the one energy that is expressing itself in many forms. Therefore, it is essential that you create a ritual that feels right for you. When it all comes down to it, we don't need any tools at all. We can simply go outside and sit with a plant and connect; we can call on the spirit of a plant to be with us when we are creating with it. Don't get caught up on the whole ritual part of the process.

Once we get out of our mind and stop thinking about the process from a limited human being point of view, we realise there are no boundaries. However, when you are first starting out, the ritual serves an important part in your connection. It helps us understand that we need to be present, we need to call upon the plant spirit, we must have focus, intent and respect. We also need to make the time to work with the plant spirit and make our concoctions. All of these are encompassed in a ritual and that's why they are so powerful.

Obviously, you don't need to go 'full ritual' on every step, so you want to start from the beginning.

When harvesting, you need to ask the plant for its permission to take a part of it and also to ask for its healing and/or wisdom. State your intention to the plant to let it know what you intend to do with it. Feel if it is ok to harvest it and, if not, leave it be.

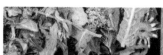

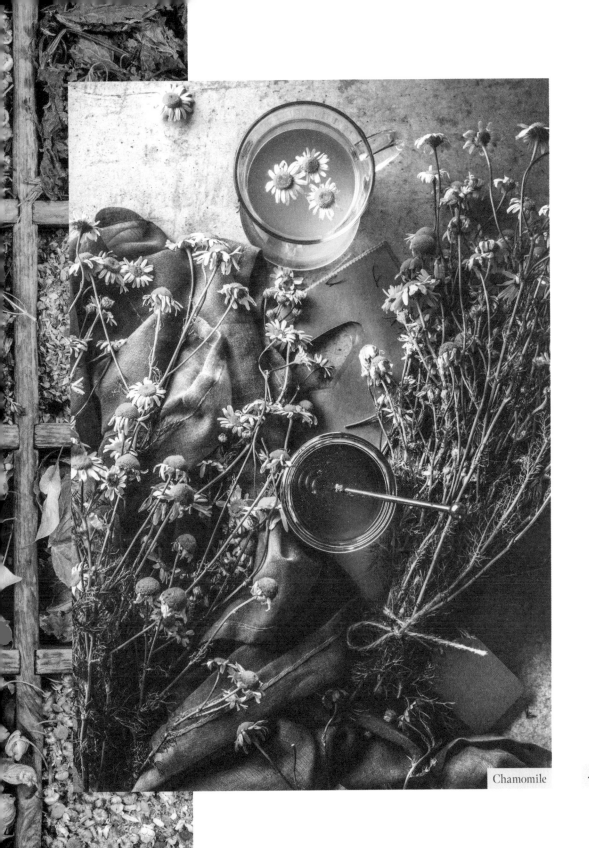

Chamomile

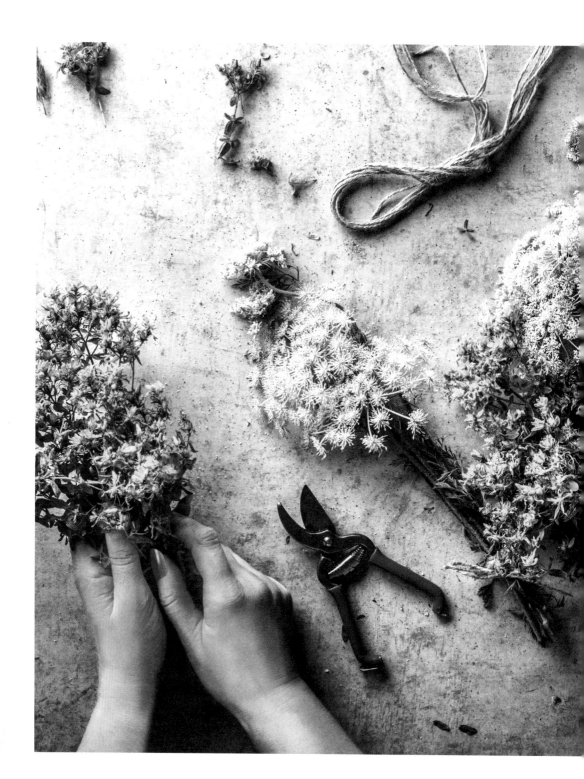

You must only take what you need. Do not strip it bare; leave enough for it to be able to recover from. If there's not enough for you to make what you need, find another avenue. We need to remember that we are working with the plant spirit, so we don't need the large amounts we might need if we were making therapeutic products.

Leave an offering. This can be as simple as giving it your gratitude. A common offering is tobacco in some countries, but only use offerings that are organic and biodegradable etc. Some water at the base of the plant is another good offering or taking away rubbish that may have been left there. I always wondered why it was important to give an offering – I mean, plants don't really need anything, right? Think of it as an energy exchange, since you are taking something from it. I tend to send my love as my gift.

We've already discussed the need to ask the plant for permission and its healing. It's important to do the Tree of Life exercise before interacting with the plant. You want to be able to sense if it is ok to harvest or use it.

If you are using dried plant matter you have bought you might like to sit with it for a while and again ask it for permission. Begin by calling the plant spirit to the dried matter in front of you. You could say something like this:

> *'I call the spirit of the* (**insert plant name here**) *to please be here with me. I ask for your healing, your guidance and wisdom. I ask that you may come back to your physical body to help with healing and guiding others.' Sit for a while and see if you feel a shift at all to know that spirit is there. Then at the end say, 'I respect and honour you. Thank you.'*

When I am creating a plant extraction, which I discuss in detail in the next chapter, I do a simple calling in of the plant spirit. I ask for it to imbue its healing and wisdom into what I am making. I close my eyes and wait for a sense that the plant spirit has heard me. I always get shivers.

This is my confirmation from spirit. Do not feel disheartened if you don't feel anything. This can take time. Do know that your intent and commitment to what you are doing is what's important. If you are genuine with this, the plant spirit will be there. Over time, you will get your confirmation.

Once I have my plant extraction, i.e. an infused oil, and am about to make up my product, for example a vervain salve, this is when I do my big ritual. I ensure I get out all of the tools and ingredients I need to make my product. I make a time when I won't be disturbed by anyone, and I love it to be nice and quiet. Then the ritual I would do would go something like this, but feel free to create your own. It has to resonate with you:

- **I cleanse the space** with a smudge stick or room spray or with Tibetan bells. I also smudge/cleanse myself.

- **I do the Tree of Life exercise** to ensure I am grounded, and then I call in the elements of the four directions: north, east, south and west. I say: 'Guardians of the north, the elementals of fire, I please ask you to be with me, to guide me, to teach me, so that I may guide and teach.' Use what feels right for you and the elements will also be placed on the directions relative to where you live i.e. south will be fire in the northern hemisphere etc. There is no right or wrong way with this as the elements are everywhere. For the southern hemisphere, I use north/fire, east/water, south/earth, west/air. I also call through the Great Spirit from above and Mother Earth from below.

- **Next, I call on my helper spirits to please be with me.** This might be your ancestors, your guides, animal spirits etc. Then call upon the plant spirit/s of what you are working with to please be with you and infuse into your product for healing and guidance for the benefit of all. Ask them to share their wisdom, and if you have a specific intention for your product ask them to imbue this element if it is for the highest good. I generally let the plant spirit imbue what it needs to, instead of me informing it what to do – remembering that it is the teacher and helper here. Really be in the

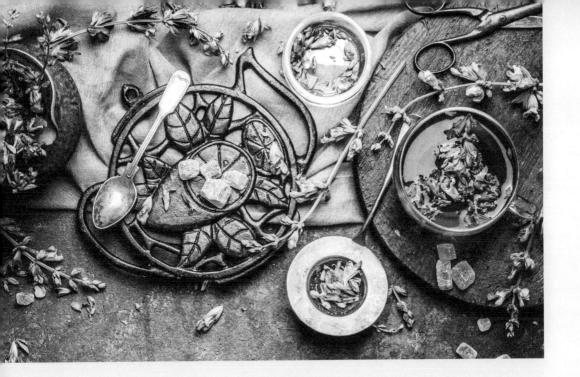

moment and feel the spirit in your workspace. If you don't feel anything, that's totally fine – it takes time – but know that it will be present if you come from a genuine place and are focused and respectful.

- **Take your time to create your product and pour your love and intention into it.** This should be a joyful experience, not a rushed one. Once you have created your product, thank the plant spirits for their help. Thank all the spirits you have called to your workspace and bid them farewell. Give your thanks to the Great Spirit, Mother Earth and the four elements/directions. Clean up and place your product in a place that is also respected. Don't just place it in a cupboard filled with junk. Everything needs to be done in a respectful manner.

There you have it. The ritual or process doesn't need to be complicated. I do mine in this manner because this aligns with my shamanic practices, and shamanic practices are universal. As you can see they are pretty simple, and you'll find that many spiritual practices encompass these anyway.

Not everyone will resonate with this method and there really is no right or wrong way. Intent is always the key with anything. Make it your own, experiment and have fun!

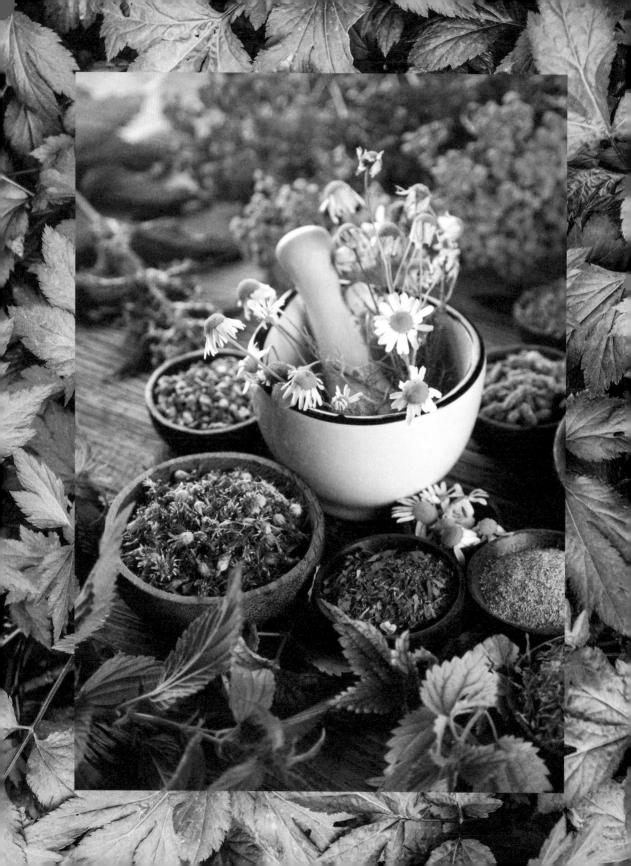

CHAPTER 5

Plant extraction methods

N ow we've reached the fun part of the book! The DIY section. This is where you will find everything you need to get started with basic Plant Spirit Medicine making. First we will look at the different methods for plant extraction, then once we have our extractions we can make products from them. The extraction methods really don't change and you will see information that is varied on how long you should leave them to extract, but there really is no hard and fast rule as every plant is different. Trust your intuition and back up what you do with research.

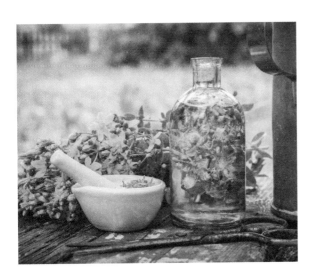

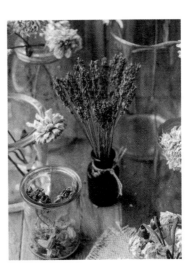

Measuring tools

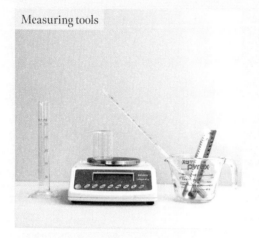

Filtering tools

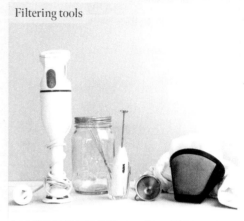

Mortars and pestles

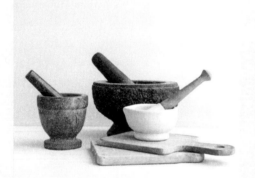

Yoghurt maker

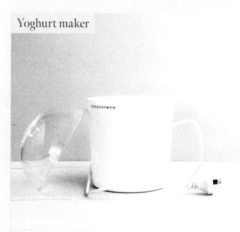

Slow cooker

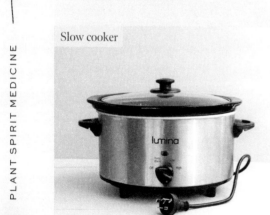

Pressure cooker

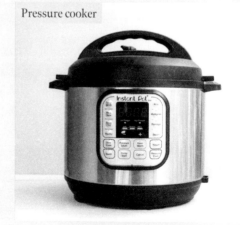

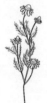

Tools

You can start basic Plant Spirit Medicine making with items already in your kitchen. It all depends on what you decide to make. I recommend starting with the minimal requirements until you get familiar with everything and have made a few products. It's easy to get carried away with wanting everything to start with, but you don't want to waste unnecessary money. Keep it simple and grow when you are more confident.

My staple items

Measuring:

- **Kitchen scales** – I have to .00 increments, but something in grams will get you started.

- **Pyrex jugs** – small and medium sizes.

- **Glass beakers** – these are really handy to have. I have four small 40 ml ones, which I use to weigh out or make small amounts of products as testers. They can also be used to heat oils/butters in, making them great all-rounders.

- **Glass measuring cylinders** – again, great to measure out quantities, but these are not necessary. You can't heat these like the glass beakers, so they can only be used as measuring tools.

- **Thermometers** – these are candy thermometers. They are important if you are making creams and anything with oils. You can also use them to stir your products while checking the temperatures.

- **Pipettes** – I use glass. These are great for measuring out drops of botanicals/essential oils but aren't really necessary as most bottles have dripolators in them for this purpose.

Filtering:

- **Muslin cloth** – especially useful for straining your plant matter from oil/water etc. Very cheap to buy from most fabric stores.

Coffee filters – again for straining your herbs/resins through. You can get metal or paper ones.

Labels – these are a must. It is so important to label your products. It's easy to forget what's in a jar or when you made something. Make this a basic practice that you do with everything. I use chalk labels and craft labels. Chalk ones are great because they can be reused over and over, but you can also just use paper and sticky tape.

Stick blender – not absolutely necessary unless you are making creams. Stick blenders are cheap and easy to pick up.

Mason jars – small and medium. These for me are a must. I always store my dried herbs in glass jars and make herbal oils in the Mason jars and keep them stored in the cupboard for future use. I also keep them preserved with vitamin E so the oils don't go rancid. Start with some small ones to house your testers and work up to larger ones once you gain confidence, otherwise you might make up a large batch of something that you might not use.

pH strips – if you intend to make creams or water-based products to go on the skin, you will need these.

Funnels – these are great for pouring your creams and oils into bottles.

Mini whisk/electric whisk – perfect for mixing up trial batches of products.

Grinding:

Mortars and pestles – there really is something special about these. They take us back to our roots. Even though I have blenders and grinders, I do pull out the mortar and pestle to work with my herbs where I can.

Handy:

Slow cooker – this isn't necessary, but it's a great tool for making herbal oils as you can use it as a water bath.

Yoghurt maker – this isn't necessary either, but it's a great tool for making herbal oils.

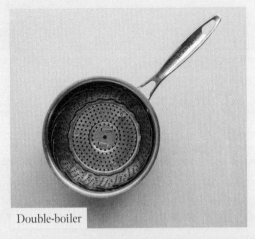

Double-boiler

A double-boiler
is also referred to
as a water bath
or bain-marie

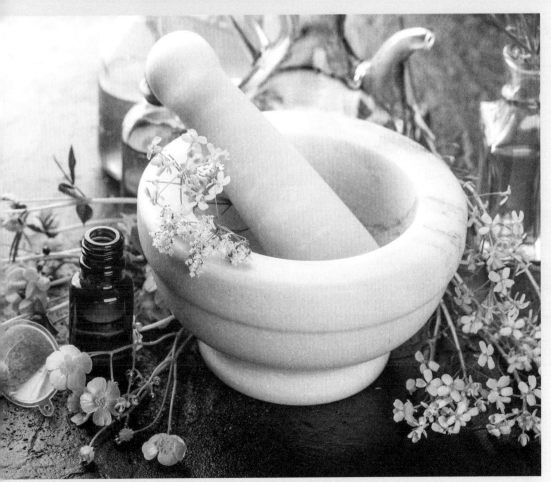

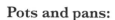

Pots and pans:

Stainless-steel pots – please don't use aluminium.

Vegetable steamers – these are perfect to create a double-boiler–type bain-marie.

Double-boiler – a double-boiler is also referred to as a water bath or bain-marie. Essentially we just need to have our glass jars/jugs not touching the bottom of the pan as it boils because the heat can be too much for them or the ingredients we are using. What we want to do is raise them off the bottom by placing either a vegetable steamer, mesh or rack to lift them up and allow the water to still flow around them.

Electrics:

Blenders – you can use large or small blenders depending on what you are making. I use a Thermomix, stick blender and Nutribullet depending on my needs. Although if you are using resins or roots, invest in something strong as you will wreck your blades or machine on too hard a material. If you get serious about your medicine making you can purchase a hammer mill grinder, which is used for Chinese Herbal Medicine grinding.

Little essentials:

Notebook – this is an essential item. Everything you do and make should be recorded in this book. This allows you to be able to replicate something that works well or fix something that didn't. You might think you will be able to remember things, but take my word for it, no matter how good your memory is there will be things that are forgotten. Make comments on how things looked, behaved or turned out. Go back to it if something happened a few days, weeks or months later that you will need to go back and fix if you create it again. In no time you'll end up with a handy book of your own making full of recipes, ideas and trials.

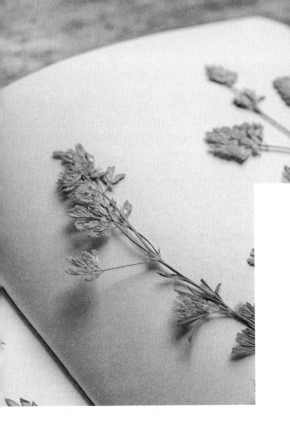

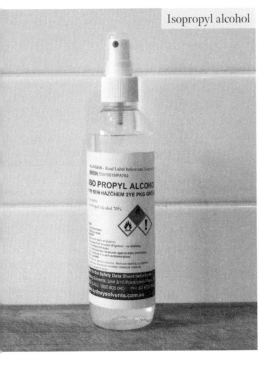

Isopropyl alcohol

Cleaning your equipment

It is vital that you keep your tools clean at all times so you don't contaminate your products, allowing mould or bacteria to grow. Ideally, you should keep all your tools dedicated to plant medicine making separate from your general cooking items.

I like to put what I can through the dishwasher to give them a good clean. Getting some 70% isopropyl alcohol/rubbing alcohol in a spray bottle and some paper towels for cleaning your items and workspace is also a good idea.

Obviously, the cleanliness of your equipment is extremely important. You should always avoid putting your fingers into your products or ingredients, as this introduces bacteria that can spoil your products and ingredients.

When cleaning your equipment after using waxes and hard butters, use paper towels to wipe out your pyrex jugs as soon as you have poured your product into jars, because when it sets it's hard to get your jugs clean again without a bit of elbow grease. Add a little detergent and boiling water to clean them out and put them in the dishwasher.

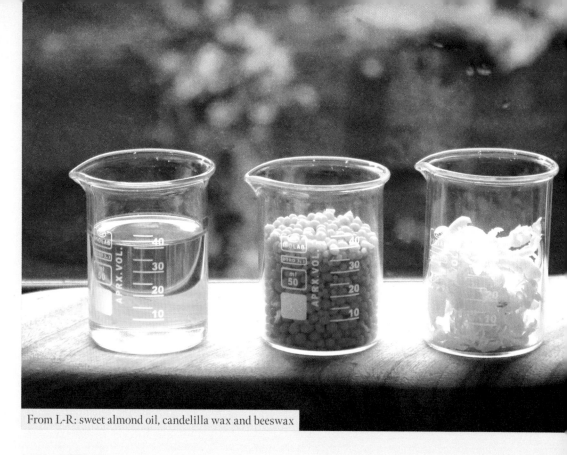

From L-R: sweet almond oil, candelilla wax and beeswax

Ingredients

Your ingredients list will depend on the products you decide to make, however, I always keep the following few items on hand because I make a lot of infused oils and salves. I'm sure you will too once you get started, as these are the most popular products to make.

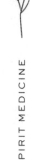

- **Sweet almond oil** – this is my favourite oil to use when making herbal oils. It doesn't have an overpowering smell and it has a light colour, so when your oil is infused you can clearly see it. It is a good stable oil at reasonable heat and is very moisturising to the skin. You can use olive oil, sunflower or other oils that you prefer. Keeping one on hand simplifies things for me.

- **Beeswax or candelilla wax** – I make a lot of balms, so I always keep candelilla wax on hand. This is a plant-based wax with a similar consistency to beeswax. Vegans prefer not to use beeswax, so it is up to you which one you would like to work with.

Alcohol – this is not necessary, but vodka is great for extracting some constituents out of plants or for preserving an essence. I have ethanol on hand, which is near pure alcohol, but it's not easy or sometimes even legal to obtain. As I am a herbalist it's available to me, but you will need to check the laws in your country. Vodka is a great all-rounder, as it is usually 40% alcohol and 60% water, which is a good ratio for extracting herbal constituents.

Vitamin E – this is an antioxidant that will ensure your oil products don't go rancid too quickly.

Herbal extraction methods

There are quite a few ways of extracting properties from a herb or plant. You need to decide first what you want to make with it. Will it be a balm, a room spray, something edible? Once you consider what you might want to make, you can then decide on the right extraction method. For instance: I want to make a salve, which is oil and wax, therefore I need to make an infused oil with my herb/plant first, and then I'll add the wax later to create the salve. If I am making a cream, which is water based, I could consider making an infusion or glycerite. If something edible, I could also do an infused oil, glycerite, oxymel or just dry my herbs first.

There really are only a few methods, so don't be too concerned. Once you make a couple you will quickly get the hang of it; I suggest you make extra small batches to start with so you don't waste any ingredients. This helps you understand the process, and when you understand what you are doing you can get more adventurous.

Labelling

Labelling is extremely important for a few reasons:

> You know what is in your bottle, so there is no mistake what you are taking.

> You know how old something is.

It's amazing how quick you can forget what is in a bottle and when you made it. Trust me, I have made this mistake many times, and to be safe I have just had to throw things out, which is such a waste.

Every label should contain the following information:

What's in your bottle – every ingredient, whether herb, water, alcohol etc. if used. Use the scientific name and common name, i.e. dandelion (*Taraxacum officinale*).

Ratios of plant to liquid (for tinctures, oils).

Date created – it's also good to add the date of when it should be ready or mark your calendar.

Fresh herb vs dried

You can make most herbal products using either fresh or dry, so what's the difference?

Fresh

Fresh herb has water in it. This not only bulks up the size of the herb, making it need more liquid to cover it if infusing it, but because of the high water content it is hard to make a strong infusion.

Water creates an environment for mould and bacteria to grow in, thus requiring a preservative.

If you are using alcohol and water as a solvent, you need to take into consideration the water content already in the plant, which can be inaccurate.

Fresh still has life force in it, and this may be exactly what you want to use.

Dried

Less solvent is needed to cover dried herb due to the lack of water content and reduces the mould or bacteria that can grow in your end product, depending on how you extract it.

Dried plants store well under the right conditions, so can be on hand when needed.

Dried herb can be ground down to a powder to be used in many different applications, making it easier to extract properties due to the low surface area of the plant.

Dried herb can require heating and shaking to allow the solvent into it to help the extraction.

It's ok to use bought dried herbs for your Plant Spirit Medicine, but I find it vitally important to get good-quality, organic herbs wherever possible. The plant spirit or life force can be completely absent from herbs that have been treated poorly. The more in tune you become with your herbs, the more you will feel if they are ok or not. In my experience with shamanism, you can call the spirit of nearly anything back to its physical part. For instance, you can call the spirit of an animal or bird back to a part of its physical body, like a bone or a feather etc. When I create wands or smudge fans, I can call back to the wood or the feathers the spirit that is attached to it. The physical object is not just a 'thing'; it becomes a vessel for the spirit to find its way to you. So for my vervain experiment I bought dried vervain and called the vervain spirit to that space in time when I created a drink from it. I got clear shivers all over me when I felt it arrive.

Harvesting and drying herbs

Picking and drying your own herbs really is a lot of fun. Not only do you get the satisfaction of acquiring a nice little stash of herbs that essentially cost you nothing, you become very attached to your herbs because you have formed a relationship with them. If you have grown them yourself, it is even more rewarding as you have nurtured them and watched them grow. Harvesting them is exciting and then having them hanging from your ceiling or on a drying rack permeates the room with their energies. This used to be a process that was a part of our lives; sadly it is not so much now. It is another reason why we have become so disconnected from the land and nature.

… having them hanging from your ceiling or on a drying rack permeates the room with their energies

When you harvest a plant, you need to respectfully gather it. This requires tuning in to the plant and asking permission from it to harvest it. You then need to leave your offering. Also, you must ensure you do no harm to the plant and only take what you need. Use something sharp to cut your pieces off as you do not want to rip or tear the plant in a way that may potentially allow disease into it.

Always ensure that you pick your herbs when there is no dew or water on them. This added water can be enough to let mould grow on them while drying. If fresh harvesting them to make into a tincture or infused oil, you might like to let it wilt for 24 hours to allow for some of the water to evaporate. Do not wash your harvest before drying it; just give it a shake to get rid of any dirt or bugs. Roots may be washed to remove dirt, but then let the outside dry before using them.

So what are the best methods for drying herbs?

Dehydrator: this is quick and good for climates where it's near impossible to dry your herbs before they go mouldy. You can also place them in the oven on a very low temperature with the door slightly open for a couple of hours. The time will always vary depending on what you drying out, so check regularly!

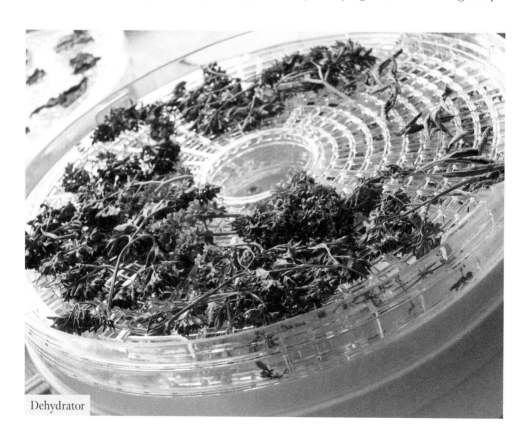
Dehydrator

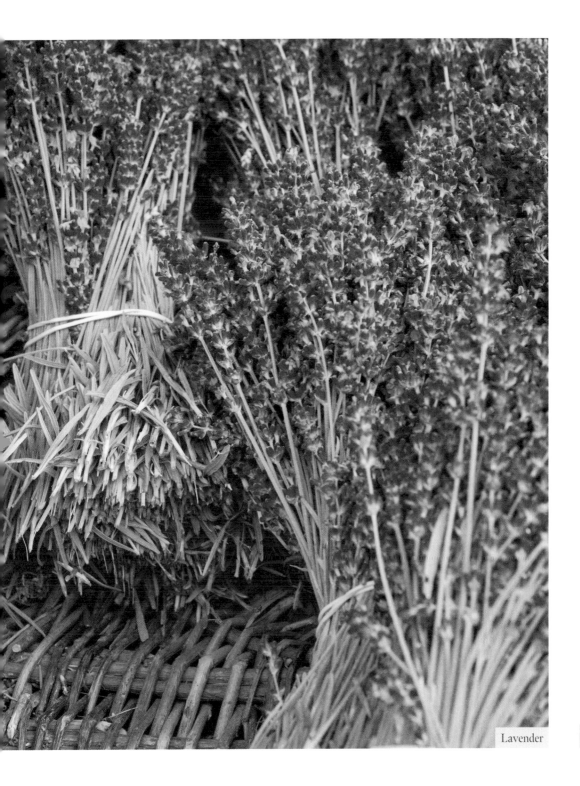

Lavender

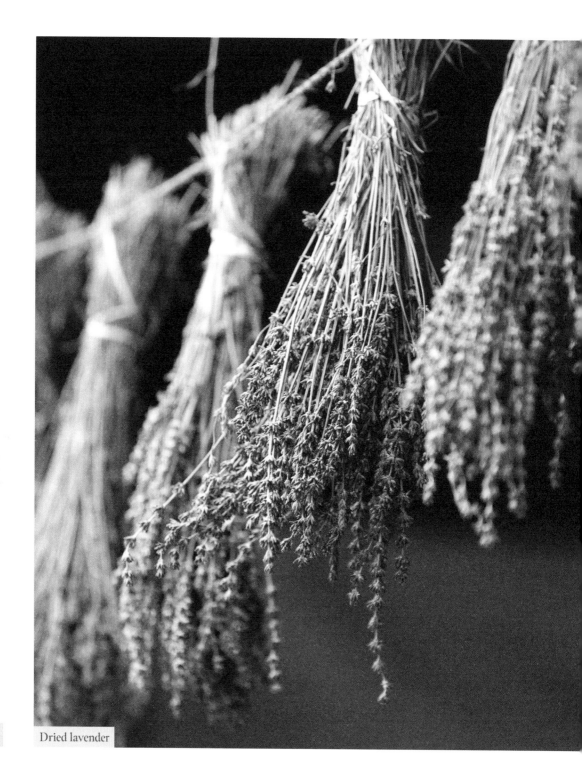

Dried lavender

- **Drying rack:** these are really handy and come in all manner of shapes and sizes. You can have layers of different herbs on different shelves. You can also make a makeshift drying screen from an old screen window. The main idea is that the plant matter has airflow, which allows them to dry fast and therefore not allowing mould to form. Placing them near a fire in cold weather is great or on top of an oil heater as long as the rack is not made of a material that will melt. This is one way I have dried out slices of ginger to be used in Chinese herbal preparations.

- **Hanging herbs:** another great way to dry herbs, which you might have seen before, is tying small amounts of the stalks together and hanging them upside down in bunches. Pot hanging racks are great for this, or you can string up a line to hang them from. Some herbs can be harder to dry, like comfrey. It has large leaves, and these sometimes go brown which is not what we want. A simple trick to hang and dry them is to thread them along a piece of cotton individually by the stalk. This gives them the airflow they need with nothing touching them.

It can be hard to tell if you've dried your plants out completely, and there's nothing worse than thinking they are, putting them in a jar and finding them mouldy later when you go to use them. Your plant is usually dry when it is very brittle and the leaves crumble when you crush them in your hand.

> **TIP:** *Place a small amount in a jar and place in the sun. If moisture forms on the inside of the glass you still have some moisture content in your plant.*

Straining and discarding your herbs

There are many ways to strain your herbs, and it all depends which process you used as an extraction method. The type of liquid you use also dictates your straining method.

- You can make simple *infusions* in a *coffee plunger or teapot with an inbuilt filter*, which allows you to strain your herb well.

- *Decoctions and infused oils* take a little more work, and muslin cloth works well in this instance. It's cheap to buy and lasts ages. Strain your mix into a Pyrex jug, by placing the muslin loosely over the jug, ensuring it can't fall into the jug once you pour your herb mix onto it. Depending on the size of your jug, you can secure it with a rubber band or place a mesh strainer underneath to support it. Pour your mix over the muslin and allow the fluid to pass through into the jug. Once most of it has dripped through, wrap the plant matter up in the muslin and tie it nice and tight. Squeeze the bundle as hard as you can to get as much liquid as possible out of it. Some people use a wine press to get the maximum yield.

- If you have ground your plant matter to a *powder*, muslin won't work as the powder will just flow straight through it. *Coffee papers* are great for this, but be mindful this can be a lengthy process. It can take a few hours, so plan ahead. Paper coffee filters can also get clogged. This happens as the plant matter settles at the bottom. You can try and pull some of it out or mix it around, but the filters are also very delicate when wet so can break. If it's clogged and you see nothing dripping out of it, change the filter. You can also buy *metal coffee strainers,* which are also great. You'll definitely need this if you are using resins.

TIPS

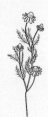

- *If you heat your oil before straining, it will strain easier.*

- *Glycerine by itself is very hard to strain through a paper filter, but if it has water content it will be quicker. I would recommend muslin cloth for anything glycerine.*

- *It's very important to discard your plant matter in a respectful way. I even discard my woodworking shavings the same way. Tossing it in the bin where it goes to landfill does not respect any spirit. I always put it in the garden somewhere and thank it for its help. If you can't do it straight away, have a little bin where you can collect everything and put it out when it's more convenient. You can also use a compost bin for anything that is able to go in it.*

Storing your herbs

Once you have your dried herbs, you need to store them in glass jars if possible. Keep them away from direct light and keep them as intact as possible, only crumbling up the leaves as you need them to ensure the highest quality. Make sure you label what's in the jar and include the date you placed them in there.

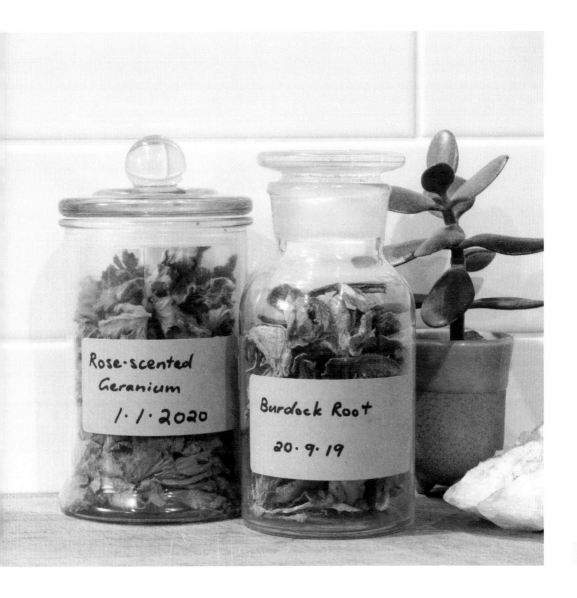

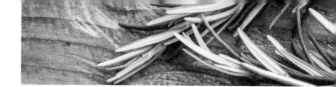

Preservation

Preserving your products is a must if you are to give them to someone or want them to last. Bacteria and mould like to grow in any product that has water or plant matter in it and can cause serious infections if you are not careful. There is a lot of confusion as to the best methods of preservation. First thing to know is that if your product contains water, it will need a preservative. If it is a product that potentially water will get into, then add a preservative. If your product is made of only oils and butters, you will need an *antioxidant*. An antioxidant prevents your oils from going rancid over time. So remember this:

Water = preservative
Oil = antioxidant
Water and oil = preservative and antioxidant

Antioxidants are easy to find and use. I use vitamin E mainly for my products, but you can use grapefruit seed or rosemary CO^2 extract. All of these are generally available in most places. Grapefruit seed extract, or citrus seed extract as it is also known, is sometimes used as a preservative but this is debatable. It is said to have antibacterial, antimicrobial and antifungal properties. It has indeed shown this in the lab, but more tests are required to confirm this is true for use in products and on the body at this time. I used grapefruit seed extract for decades in my own skincare products and have never had an issue with bacteria or mould, however, now that I sell on a commercial scale I use a preservative that is known for its broad-spectrum activity.

Preservatives are a little harder to come to terms with. We want something completely natural – I get it. There is always going to be someone that cannot tolerate your preservative, so keep this in mind, but generally these people are already aware that they react to certain products. Some people just are highly sensitive to anything on their skin.

I always use preservatives that are approved for organic skincare. Naticide® is a popular one as it is very effective, however, it does have a strong almond smell. This doesn't worry many people, but it can overpower the smell of your product. You only need to add up to 1% to your product and it actually has to be listed on your label as parfum or fragrance, because the name is trademarked. I use another one called

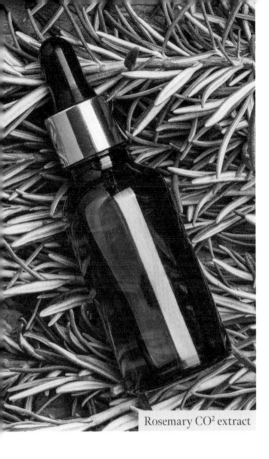
Rosemary CO² extract

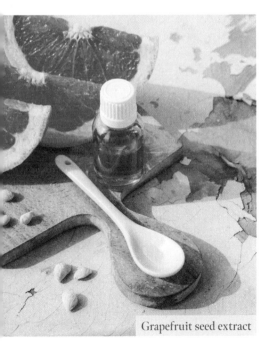
Grapefruit seed extract

Plantaserv M. It is also a broad-spectrum preservative that is very effective and the smell is less potent than Naticide. The preservative is derived from natural sources such as pine, rowan and willow. It has many names around the world and is sometimes known as Preservative Eco, Geogard ECT or Mikrokill ECT. Another good one that has been recommended to me is Liquid Germall Plus. There are many other options for natural preservatives, so you need to find what is available in your country and research how effective it is and what it is mainly used for.

Also keep in mind that you can purchase preservatives for anhydrous products (meaning a product that contains no water). Why would we use one if it has no water? Because at some stage it may come into contact with water. It is used as a precaution and needs to be oil soluble because it is added to oils.

One thing you need to be aware of is preservatives work best between certain pH ranges, so it is important to test your product's pH before adding the preservative and also after. This is why so many people opt to make products that have no water in them, thus only requiring an antioxidant. Once you get a hang of the whole pH testing part, though, you can make amazing products. We'll touch more on this when we get to cream making.

Infusions/decoctions

Most of you will be familiar with infusions already if you've ever made yourself a cup of tea. It's as simple as infusing your herb in boiling water. The general rule is about 30 g of herb to 600 ml of water. I tend to just use a teaspoon of herb to one small cup of water for any tea that I make from fresh herb. If you need it strong, then obviously make it more concentrated. Eye baths of chamomile tea or calendula are good ones here. Just let your herb or teabag steep for 15 minutes, let cool and then dab some on your eye with something soft and absorbent. Infusions are also good to use as the water element of a cream, which we will cover later.

A decoction is when you bring herbs to a simmer in a pot for around 15 to 30 minutes. Soaking in warm water for 10 minutes prior can also enhance the decoction. This method is normally used for more dense herbs, like roots and twigs. Chinese Herbal Medicine relies on a similar method and it is extremely powerful, so don't underestimate how beneficial this process is. I have a Chinese electric herb pot, and there's something magical about brewing up my herbs in it. You can buy one you can just place on your cooktop, or you can use an electric one that plugs in like a normal jug. It depends on what you can afford. You can also use a stainless-steel pot – just don't use aluminium.

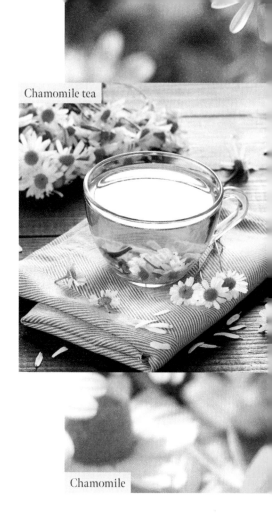

Chamomile tea

Chamomile

I tend to just use a teaspoon of herb to one small cup of water for any tea that I make from fresh herb

METHOD:

If using a Chinese herb jug:

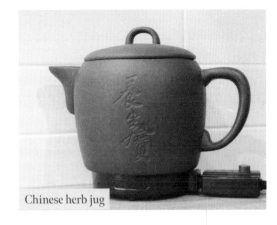

Chinese herb jug

- *Place your herbs in the pot and cover with warm water. Delicate herbs or flowers are normally placed in near the end of the boil, whereas roots and twigs would go in first as they take longer. Let sit for about 10 minutes first and then bring to the boil.*

- *Simmer until about half the liquid has evaporated. Strain and put this liquid aside.*

- *Repeat the first steps, strain and add this new liquid to the first lot.*

- *Repeat once more, and again add the last of the liquid to the first lot.*

This method ensures maximum extraction of all constituents and makes a strong decoction.

Infusions and decoctions don't have to be taken internally. You can use them on the skin, eyes, hair, in baths or even in spritzer bottles for room sprays etc.

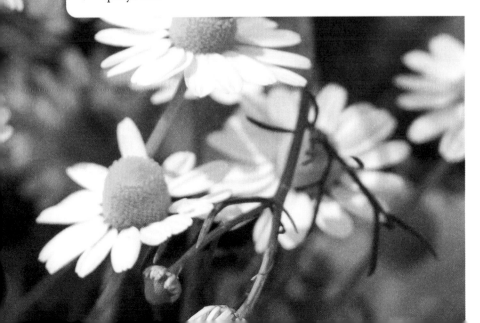

Macerations

Maceration is the name given to infusing plant material in a solvent or menstruum, i.e. water/alcohol/oil/vinegar etc., over a period of usually a couple of weeks. These include tinctures, infused oils, oxymels and glycerites.

Tinctures/liquid extracts

Tinctures and liquid extracts are a preferred method of extraction for many reasons. They are made with a solvent of alcohol and water. The percentage of alcohol to water varies depending on the make-up of the plant and what constituents need to be extracted. For Plant Spirit Medicine we will focus on a mix of 40% alcohol to 60% water (you can use vodka), as the detail on extraction percentages is a big topic and not needed for this work.

Tinctures generally have a good success rate of extracting both the alcohol and water-soluble ingredients. The alcohol also serves as a preservative, which can make tinctures last for many years. Tinctures are concentrated and easily absorbed. They can be added into creams or solely used by themselves. They can be taken internally and used externally. If the alcohol is a worry for you, just before you use it you can delicately boil some of the alcohol from it. The difference between a liquid extract and a tincture is generally only the ratio of herb to alcohol/water. Liquid extracts will be 1:1– 1:2 and tinctures are anything over 1:3.

As a herbalist, I use near pure ethanol for this process. If you are able to acquire some, you generally need to add water to bring the alcohol percentage down. If you are making a tincture from calendula, which needs 90% alcohol, this is fine, but there are not too many herbs that require such a high content – generally, just resinous herbs. You can make a calendula-infused oil from any percentage alcohol;

> Fresh plant matter will have water content, which will throw out your ratio of alcohol to water

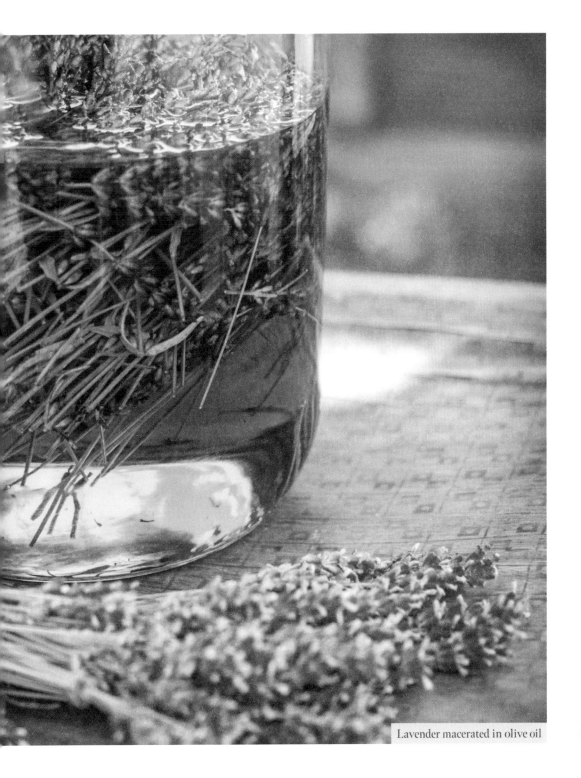

Lavender macerated in olive oil

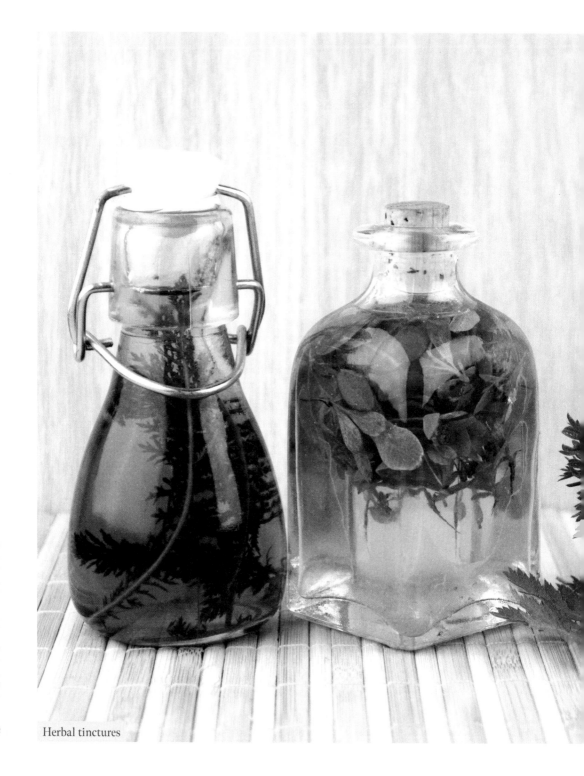

Herbal tinctures

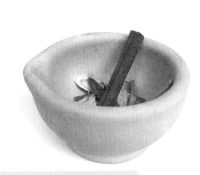
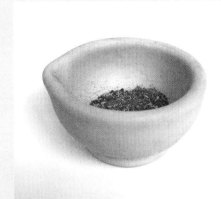

Dried licorice and cinnamon

just know that maximum extraction happens at 90%. Infusing calendula without alcohol first into an oil is also not very effective.

If you want to be accurate in your tincture making, you can obtain a copy of the *British Herbal Pharmacopoeia* or one that pertains to your country. The British one covers many herbs we commonly use, and they give you the percentages of alcohol to water needed to extract the constituents of each herb efficiently. The pharmacopoeias can be quite pricey, but you can pick up older versions that still have a lot of useful information in them. Keep in mind, though, as we are making Plant *Spirit* Medicine, that you shouldn't be too concerned about the exact science, but if you are a qualified herbalist this is important information.

You can use either fresh or dried plant matter for this process, however, I would suggest using dry herbs to get started. Fresh plant matter will have water content, which will throw out your ratio of alcohol to water. If you want to use fresh herb, you might want to create a glycerite using glycerine instead. Glycerites are discussed later in this chapter.

METHOD:

It's important to break the plant down as much as possible to allow for the alcohol/water mix to penetrate it.

A mortar and pestle is great for this, or you can place it in a blender with the alcohol/water mix. I'm making a fluid extract for this example.

The process is exactly the same as a tincture; just the liquid ratios to herbs are different.

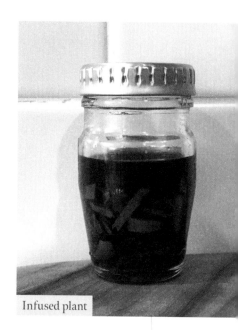

Infused plant

- *First weigh how much plant matter you have. Decide on whether you want to make a 1:1 or higher, which means one part herb to one part alcohol/water mix. I made a 1:6 as I needed more liquid to be able to cover my chunky herbs.*

- *I decided to make a small jar to see what it was like before making something bigger. The finer you can get your dried herbs the better, as when it is bulky it will take more liquid to cover it. My plant mix weighed 7 g and I made an alcohol/water mix of 40% alcohol and 60% water, which equalled 42 g in total.*

- *Place the plant into a jar and cover with the alcohol/water. You can use vodka as this is readily available everywhere and has a good alcohol/water ratio. Brandy can also be used. Ensure the plant material is thoroughly covered. If you intend to make them medicinal, you will need to consult a pharmacopoeia to find out the correct ratio of alcohol/water and calculate the water content in your plant if you are using fresh plant.*

- *Make sure that when you are working with the plant you talk to it, asking for its healing to be in-stowed into your mix. Sometimes you will get a feeling or shivers to know that the plant spirit is indeed with you.*

- *You need to leave the mix for 14 days, shaking it vigorously three times a day if possible. Every time you pick it up to shake it, connect with the plant spirit. Make it a habit of connecting as much as possible. Keep it in a warm place, but not too hot. If you are using a high per cent alcohol, do not leave it in the sun or the heat.*

- *Ensure you label it as discussed earlier.*

- *After 14 days, strain, discard the plant matter, place the liquid in an amber glass bottle and store away from heat and light. This is now your finished product, so ensure you label it again when strained with what's in it etc. You can leave it for a lot longer if there is bark or root in it. Keep checking on it from time to time to see how strong it gets.*

Infused wines/alcohol

There are many infused types of wine that have been used over the centuries. One you might be familiar with is mulled wine. This is one of my winter favourites, full of gorgeous herbs and spices! I was super surprised to be at a café in Paris where mulled wine was on the menu, served up with fresh slices of orange. Yum! Even just your normal bottled alcohols like gin and Jägermeister have infused herbs in their formula. Alcohol helps draw medicinals into the body, so it's needless to say adding herbals makes for a highly therapeutic drink indeed. Even tinctures are medicinal alcohol infusions. You could even make a range of herbal liquors. The limits are again endless, but I won't be going into how to make these because that in itself could be

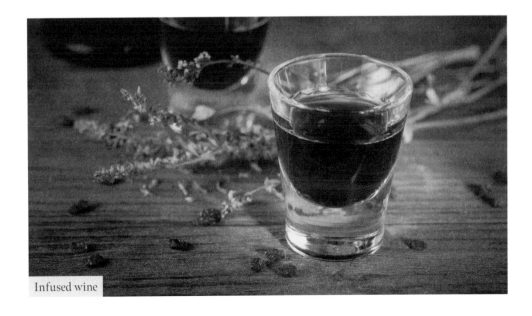

Infused wine

another book entirely and I am no expert on this topic. Another alcohol that is also good for extracting herbs is brandy if you don't want to use vodka. Brandy is a dark spirit and slightly sweet, making it a good alcohol for infusing herbs for consumption.

Medicinal wines have been used in Chinese Herbal Medicine for thousands of years. Yes, thousands. Chinese Herbal Medicine has been around for that long. Their medicinal wines included liniments for external use. They infused many herbs in a porcelain jar with a white alcohol like rice wine or plum wine, which has a high alcohol content, and would let them sit for around 10 days to three months, shaking vigorously each day. Then some would be buried in the earth for another month or up to 100 days. This would then be dug up, strained and placed in bottles to be used topically when necessary. Liniments are extremely effective for penetrating the skin because of the alcohol content and the herbs used help move the blood flow and qi to relieve the trauma. Some of their medicinal wines could also be taken internally, making them practically the same as a tincture.

However, this book is not about making therapeutics, so I will explain how I used red wine to make my vervain plant spirit concoction for myself. You don't need much wine and believe me it doesn't taste good, so there is no need to waste good wine.

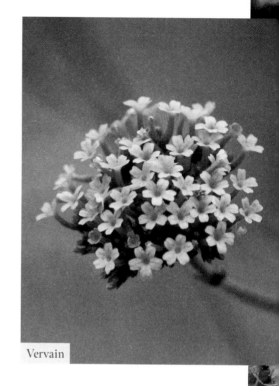

Vervain

You don't need much wine and believe me it doesn't taste good, so there is no need to waste good wine

RITUAL RECIPE:

Vervain- and rose-infused wine ritual to bring in love.

METHOD:

- *Create your ritual space by clearing your space first, performing your Tree of Life grounding exercise and calling in your helper spirits. Call upon the plant spirits of vervain and rose to be with you and infuse into your wine for your healing and guidance. Ask for them to share their wisdom, and if you are using it for love state that you wish to find love in whatever way that looks for your highest good. Really be in the moment.*

- *Add to a stainless-steel pot 50 ml of red wine, a sprinkle of vervain and rose petals (freshly grown rose if possible or organic with no pesticide use). Heat very gently; don't let it boil, just let it come to a good heat. It doesn't need to be on there long. At every moment, try and feel the plant spirits with you and infusing into your wine.*

- *Take off the heat and strain. When cooled slightly, take a sip. When you drink it, be present and savour the smell, taste and feel. Respect the process. Say to yourself or out loud, 'I attract love, I AM love.'*

- *Thank the plant spirits for their help and record everything in your notebook. Then allow the plant spirits to help you. For me this took around three months, with different experiences happening over that time until I had my 'a-ha' moment. Once that occurred my whole life began to change because I had a different perception of myself, so my outer world had to shift to match my inner.*

Rose buds

Infused oils

Infused oils are probably the most popular way to infuse plants/herbs for the home herbalist and skincare maker. They are so versatile and can be used in salves, ointments, creams and many other products. Once you start they become addictive, and in time you'll end up with a dedicated cupboard with jars of all sorts of herb oils to have on hand for your creations. They are easy to make, easy to come by the ingredients and the rewards are plenty.

You might already be familiar with infused oils for cooking, like rosemary-infused olive oil or garlic oil. These are as simple as placing your herb into a bottle of oil and ensuring the herb is completely covered (or mould can grow). Leave it for about a month and voila! You now have a herb-infused oil you can pour over salad or on your roast vegies. Yum! Obviously, you need to make sure you use edible oil and the plant you put in there is also safe to ingest.

> # Only oil-soluble constituents will be extracted from your plant matter in an oil infusion

Only oil-soluble constituents will be extracted from your plant matter in an oil infusion. When making Plant Spirit Medicine this is not an issue, because some of the physical plant will be in your finished product and that is the key here. But if you are making therapeutic products, keep this in mind. The main oils that will be extracted are the aromatic oils, volatile oils (essential oils), resins and oleoresins.

There are so many methods for creating infused oils for making natural products. It can be as simple as placing your herbs in a jar and covering them with oil, then leaving the jar in a warm or sunny place and shaking it twice a day for 10 to 14 days. There are always other methods that can be used to extract the physical constituents from the plant more effectively to use as a therapeutic oil, and I will go into these here. I use all these methods depending on what plant matter I have, the time I have available and what the most efficient extraction method is. This does take some experimenting, so always make up small amounts when first starting out. The process

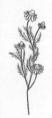

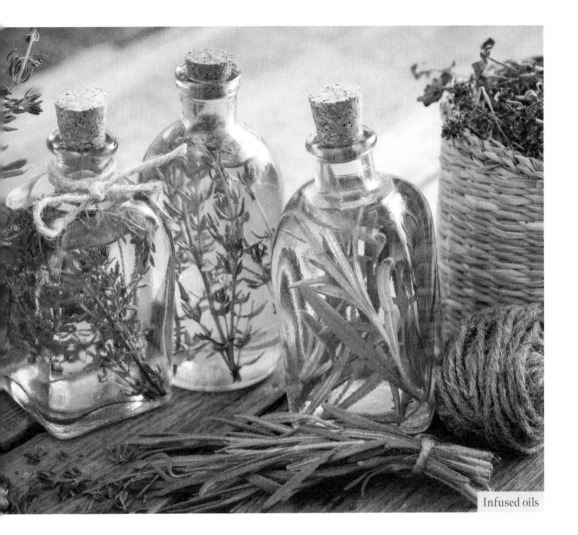

Infused oils

is not about rushing; it's about enjoying the process, enjoying the relationship building with the plant and infusing all your love and care into your products.

Always make sure that the plant matter is completely covered with a little more oil than needed so it stays well under the oil and none of it protrudes or mould will develop. Every time you give it a shake, ensure it is still completely covered. Use a chopstick or something clean to poke it back under if it pokes through. Also note that some dried herbs will absorb some oil, so you might need to add more oil to it after a day. Be sure to add this as a note in your notebook, so you can add the extra right from the beginning next time.

Heating infused oils

Throwing herbs into cold room temperature oil may not do much at all. The liquid needs to be able to permeate the plant matter, so heating the oil speeds the process up and gets it going. However, don't heat the oil too hot or for too long, as this can make it unstable, especially if you are using a delicate oil, and never let it boil. Olive oil or sweet almond oil are good for heating. Oils will also go rancid over time if exposed to heat, air and light. Any vegetable oil will do, though.

There are many types of oils available these days, so I suggest you find something either made locally or fair trade that is environmentally friendly and organic if possible. You could use olive, sweet almond, jojoba (actually a wax but still fine), coconut, macadamia, sunflower, argan, baobab etc. Just start with something within your budget that won't break the bank when you make mistakes. This is why I recommend olive and sweet almond oil to start with, but feel free to use what you like.

You can make infused oils with either fresh or dried plant material. Keep in mind that fresh plants will have water content in them and water and oil don't mix. The water content will also attract mould, but you can strain this out to a point. You might like to let your fresh plant wilt for 24 hours before using it. There are a couple of methods I would suggest when using fresh plant matter in oils. I will give you some tips on the best way to handle them after the following heating methods.

METHOD 1: HEATING WITH NATURAL SUNLIGHT

This is termed the 'folk method'. Anyone can do it and it can be very effective.

- *Grind or finely chop your plant matter.*

- *Weigh your plant matter first, then place it in your jar to around ½ to ¾ full. Write down how much herb you used in your notebook.*

- *Next, pour your oil into a measuring jug so you can measure how much you are going to put in the pot and how much is needed to cover the plant. This allows you to be able to replicate what you have made if it works out well*

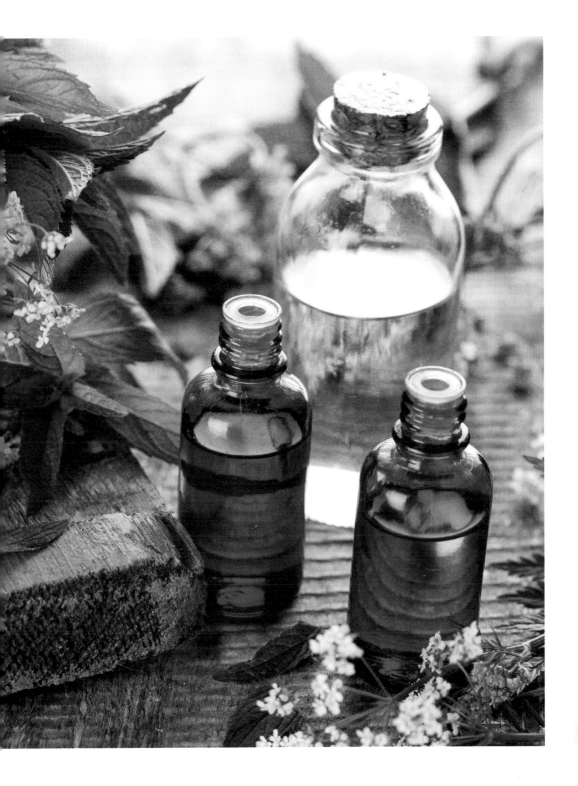

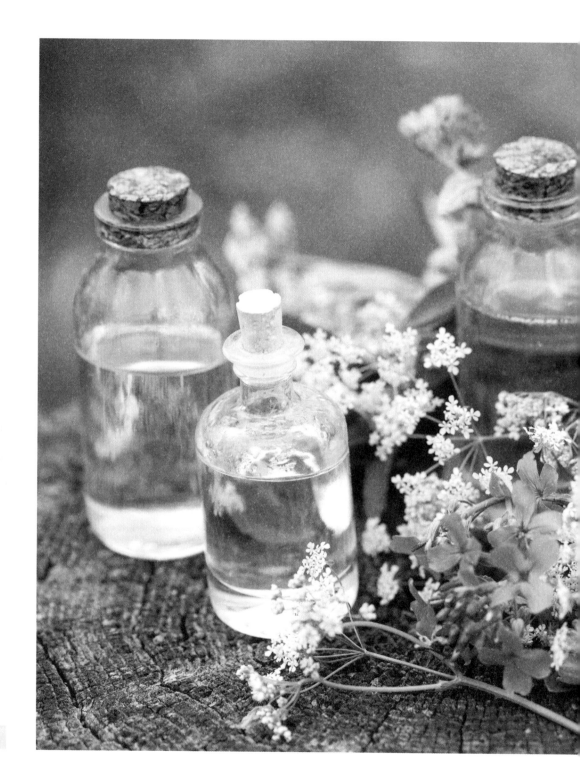

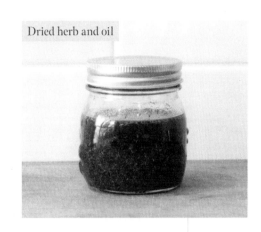
Dried herb and oil

because you now have a plant to oil ratio, i.e. 7 g of plant to 28 g of oil.

- Pour the oil over the herb in the jar and fill it to about 1.5 cm or ½ inch above the herb. Some herbs will expand in the jar once they have been in the oil for a few hours or overnight. The more oil you add above the mix the better. Write in your journal if your plant swells at all so you can allow for extra next time you make it.

- Stir or shake the jar to ensure all of the herb is covered and submerged in the oil. Tighten the lid on your jar, and then place it in a thick paper bag or some thin material so it can be kept out of direct sunlight (which can cause it to go rancid) and place somewhere warm in the sun for around 10 to 14 days. **(The only exception here is St John's wort, which requires fresh flowers and to be in direct sunlight to make its bright red oil.)** You can also place it near a heat source if there is no sun. Nothing above 38°C/100°F (approximately).

- Shake the jar a couple of times or more each day. Check to make sure the herb isn't protruding above the oil, as this can make the herb mouldy, which will affect the oil and you will need to throw it away. You can use a chopstick to push it back under the oil. Don't ever poke it down with your finger or you will introduce bacteria into your oil.

- Once the time is up, if you feel your oil is not finished you can leave it in the heat for up to three weeks. You can also strain it and add new plant material to the oil and leave again for 10 to 14 days, shaking at least twice a day, which will give you a stronger oil. You can even switch out the plant matter for another plant so it becomes a mixed oil, or place both herbs in there from the start.

- Once finished in the heat source, strain the herb, jar and label.

- Add your antioxidant when cool.

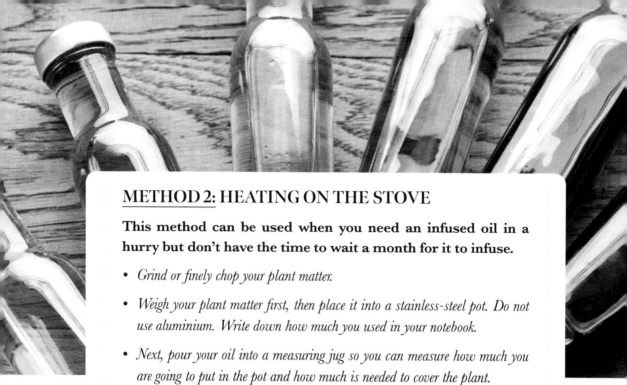

METHOD 2: HEATING ON THE STOVE

This method can be used when you need an infused oil in a hurry but don't have the time to wait a month for it to infuse.

- *Grind or finely chop your plant matter.*

- *Weigh your plant matter first, then place it into a stainless-steel pot. Do not use aluminium. Write down how much you used in your notebook.*

- *Next, pour your oil into a measuring jug so you can measure how much you are going to put in the pot and how much is needed to cover the plant.*

- *Cover the plant matter with oil and record how much oil you used.*

- *Bring the oil to a heat that is not simmering, but close to it. Oils become unstable at high heats.*

- *Generally, as soon as the oil changes colour it is ready to take off the heat. This can happen really quickly and the colour will depend on what plant you have in the oil. I find it hard to tell when the oil has changed colour because generally there is so much herb in it. Sometimes you can see it really clearly though, depending on what you use.*

- *Once off the heat you can strain this straight away, remembering that hot oil will strain well, so have this set up before you start.*

- *Jar and label.*

- *Add your antioxidant when cool.*

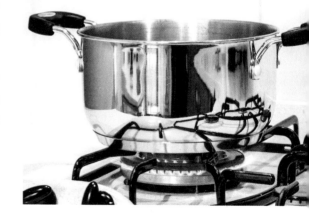

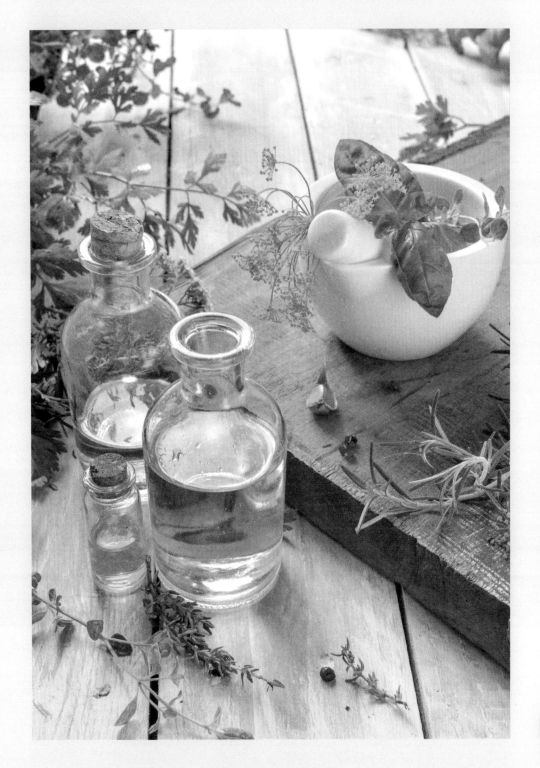

Whenever you are heating oil in a glass jar, make sure you are using proper Mason/ preserving jars . . .

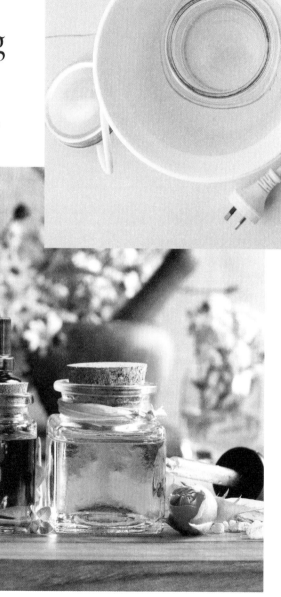

Yoghurt maker

METHOD 3: USING A YOGHURT MAKER

This is one of the methods I use often – mainly because I am forgetful in the kitchen when I have things on the stove and I like to free up my time to do the hundreds of other things I always have on the go at once. Yoghurt makers have a gentle heat, which makes them a great choice for infusing oils.

I purchased a yoghurt maker for around $50. You can use Mason jars in them to do one or a few oils at once, but I prefer to do one big batch. For this I have a coffee plunger glass insert that fits nicely into my yoghurt maker. Keep in mind that if you are using a plant for which you want to keep the volatile oils from escaping i.e. peppermint, rosemary, frankincense etc., you might want to use a Mason jar and keep the lid on or the oils will escape. *Whenever you are heating oil in a glass jar, make sure you are using proper Mason/preserving jars designed to be heated. You do not want your jar to break.*

- *Grind or finely chop your plant matter.*

- *Weigh your plant matter first, place it in your jar to around ½ to ¾ full, then write down how much you used in your notebook.*

- *Next, pour your oil into a measuring jug so you can measure how much you are going to put in the jar and how much is needed to cover the plant.*

- *Cover the plant matter with oil and record how much oil you used.*

- *Place your jar into your yoghurt maker and put the lid on. Voila – leave it to work its magic for about 10 days. You will need to stir or shake it a couple of times a day, some say every two hours. Keep an eye also on the colour and smell of your oil. If you have a yoghurt maker with a thermostat you can set it to around 38°C/100°F.*

- *Your oil should be done by the end of the 10 days. Check the colour of the oil and also check the smell.*

- *Strain with whichever method works best for your medium.*

- *Jar and label. Add your antioxidant when cool.*

METHOD 4: DOUBLE-BOILER/WATER BATH ON THE STOVE

This is a method I use regularly. This is also the method that works best for infusing resins, which I've outlined on the next page. Sometimes this is how I start my infusion to get it nice and hot, and then I transfer it to the yoghurt maker for a few days. This gives it a good start.

First of all, we need to make sure we have the right tools to create a double-boiler *(refer to the tools section on how to make your own).*

Fill the double-boiler with enough water to submerge your jar or jug in, so the water sits around the height of the materials in the jar. I find this allows the heat to distribute more evenly than just coming from the bottom. If you have an open jug with your oil, ensure when the water boils that splashes of water don't get into your oil.

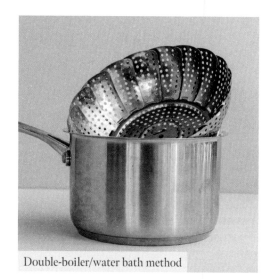

Double-boiler/water bath method

- *Grind or finely chop your plant matter.*

- *Weigh your plant matter first, place it in your jar to around ½ to ¾ full, then write down how much you used in your notebook.*

- *Next, pour your oil into a measuring jug, so you can measure how much you are going to put in the jar and how much is needed to cover the plant.*

- *Cover the plant matter with oil and record how much oil you used.*

- *Decide if you need to have the lid on or off. Volatile or essential oils will boil out if you have the lid off. As for the previous method, ensure you are using a proper Mason jar if you are going to keep the lid on, as you don't need a glass jar explosion in your kitchen. If you have fresh plant matter in your jar and are not worried about needing to hold on to any volatile oils, make sure you have no lid on your jar. This will allow for some of the water to evaporate as it heats.*

- *Bring the water up to a simmer. Keep an eye on the water as it evaporates and refill with boiling water from the jug to keep it going if it has boiled down too much.*

- *For normal plant matter, keep it in this water bath for around 15 minutes to an hour. If you are using resins, this might take up to three hours. Myrrh, for example, takes many hours. Always keep checking on your oils. Check for colour changes and the smell of your oil.* **Be careful when taking the lids off your jars to check for smell. Use a good thick towel to cover the lid. They can build up pressure and will be very hot.**

- *Once finished, strain, jar and label.*

- *Add your antioxidant when cool.*

Infusing resins

Resins generally either dissolve in oil or the oil-soluble ingredients are extracted into the oil. The kind of resin you have will determine how long it needs in the double-boiler. If it dissolves nearly straight away, take it out. If it doesn't, you might need to keep checking: a) the colour of the oil to see if it is changing and b) after carefully removing the lid with a tea-towel the smell. (But be quick so you don't let all the essential oils out! They will settle into the oil again later once it has cooled down.)

Common resins are frankincense and pine, which are especially good for pain salves. Keep in mind the sustainability and ethical issues around the farming of frankincense, as many species are becoming over-harvested. This is why I never use the essential oil. Essential oils need a crazy amount of plant matter to make and only extract the oils from the plant. Many of the other active constituents aren't drawn out of the resin/plant. This is not sustainable, especially as demand grows. The main actions are in the full resin, not just its essential oil component, so be aware of people making therapeutic claims for products that only contain essential oils dropped into a salve and where the rest of the plant constituents aren't in it. This is why it's vitally important to have the necessary training if you are going to create a business and make therapeutic claims about your products. One last point to mention is that many plant constituents work synergistically together and when you extract or isolate one particular active constituent you might get side effects. However, if you have the full plant profile with the other constituents, side effects are less likely to occur.

When straining resins, I secure a paper coffee filter over a Pyrex jug with a rubber band. A metal coffee filter can also be used. The filtering process literally takes hours and hours, but it is such a rewarding process to see your finished product and the smell will be amazing!

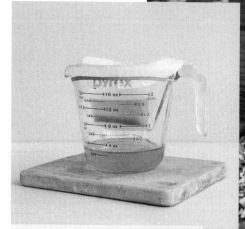

Filtering resin using coffee filter paper

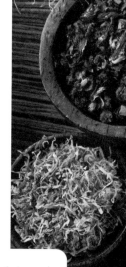

TIP: *Grind your resin. Most resins need to be ground down first before being infused in oil. The more pliable the resin, like pine or fir for example, the less you need to grind down. These may be used as they are. Place hard resins in the freezer before trying to grind them. If you can put your grinder blades in there as well, do so. Once resin gets ground too much or heated it can become sticky and is a nightmare to remove. Use a mortar and pestle if you like or you can buy resin already ground (my preference). Once ground it can lose some of its oils, so it must be stored well in a jar with a lid.*

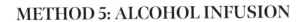

METHOD 5: ALCOHOL INFUSION

This is one of the most efficient methods of extraction and one that also has the added bonus of a little alcohol to help with the preservation of your final product.

It involves soaking your plant matter in alcohol for 24 hours before infusing in oil. The theory behind this method means that the plant matter is initially broken down with the alcohol, allowing for more of its constituents to be extracted into the oil, which wouldn't normally occur in just the oil alone. This method is what I use to make my calendula-infused oil, the recipe for which is below the following steps.

- *Grind or finely chop your plant matter.*

- *Weigh your plant matter first, place it in your jar to around ½ to ¾ full then write down how much you used in your notebook.*

- *Pour in a little vodka, just enough to wet the plant matter – you don't want it to be soaking in it, it just needs to be moist. You should be able to grab a small bunch and it not drip. Let this sit for around 24 hours.*

- *Next, pour your oil into a measuring jug so you can measure how much you are going to put in the jar and how much is needed to cover the plant.*

- *Cover the plant matter with oil and record how much oil you used.*

- *Put it all through the blender and then place the jar in a water bath with the lid off, at around 50–60°C/120–140°F. This helps to evaporate the alcohol and water. Boil it until you can't smell the alcohol in it. Leave a little alcohol in it to preserve it that little bit more and prolong its shelf life.*

- *Add your antioxidant when cool.*

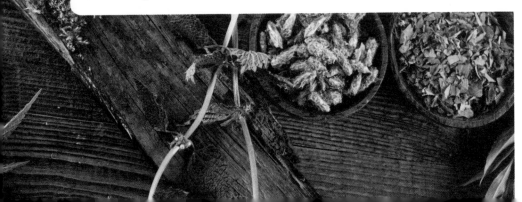

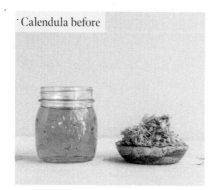

Calendula before

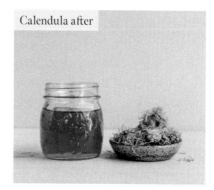

Calendula after

OIL RECIPE: CALENDULA-INFUSED OIL

Calendula has many uses internally and externally, but it also has its spiritual qualities. It is known to be protective, calming and cleansing inside and out. Being a plant that loves the sun, it is best harvested when fully open in the sunlight. Calendula therefore can also bring warmth to your being when you need it.

As mentioned previously, calendula is a popular ingredient in skincare and many home skincare makers create their own infused oil. Here is the method I use to create my oil, which extracts the constituents fully and takes approximately a day and a half. For this method I use 95% ethanol, but if you only have vodka that is still ok – just know it won't be as strong, though it will be stronger than just infusing the flowers in oil. You might also like to check out an Asian grocery store for Chinese rice wine. You can get some high percentage rice wines (sometimes 60%) for a good price.

First you need to ensure your calendula is a nice deep to mid-orange colour. Generally, if it is a light yellow it may be old.

METHOD:

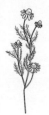

- *Blend 25 g of dried calendula to a powder. (I haven't tried it with fresh, so you might need to adjust the measurements of oil later.)*

- *Add 25 g of 95% ethanol or other alcohol (vodka) and stir to make sure it is all wet.*

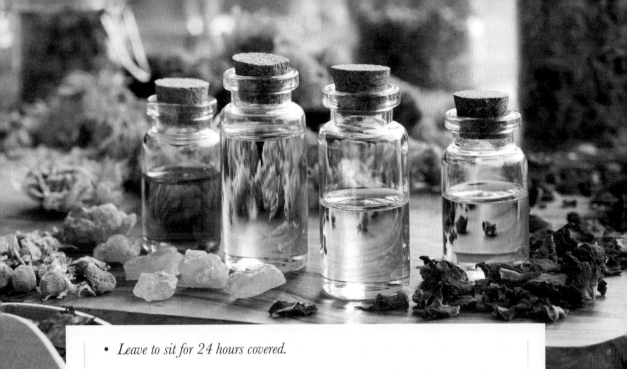

- *Leave to sit for 24 hours covered.*

- *After 24 hours, pour in around 250 g or 300 ml of an oil of your choice. I use sweet almond oil.*

- *Blend it all in a mixer or use a stick blender.*

- *Place the jar in a water bath and bring the temperature of the water up to around 50–60°C/120–140°F. Keep the lid off your jar to allow for some of the alcohol mix to evaporate off. The time will vary. When you can't smell as much alcohol or the volume has gone down, it should be ready. I leave a little alcohol in mine to preserve it a bit better, just in case. Remember that alcohol can irritate some people's skin, so if you use it in a balm make sure you boil off as much alcohol as you can before you make it. It's impossible to boil off all the alcohol, as it needs higher temperatures for a longer period of time, which obviously can damage your oil. Another reason why you shouldn't put too much in at the beginning.*

- *Strain, jar and label. If you use a powder, double over your muslin cloth when straining and use one with a tight weave.*

- *Add your antioxidant when cool. I used 2.5 g of vitamin E, which was 1% of the 250 g I had in total. You may lose some oil in the straining process, but you can add just a little more at the beginning to allow for this.*

METHOD 6: PRESSURE COOKING

This is a method I have tried, but I'm no expert on it. I find it hard to work out the times and if the oil is under too much heat etc. This is a point of confusion with pressure cooking.

Theoretically, the method heats the product extremely high but for a short period of time. I'm not sure how stable the oil is at these temperatures, so would advise using olive oil. I have made comfrey-infused oil in a pressure cooker, and it turned out really dark green and didn't smell funny so I assumed it was ok. I suggest you experiment. The Instant Pot is a widely used electric pressure cooker that can be set at low temperatures, has a stainless-steel insert and is effective for making decoctions through to syrups. You can also use it instead of a yoghurt maker to do a water bath.

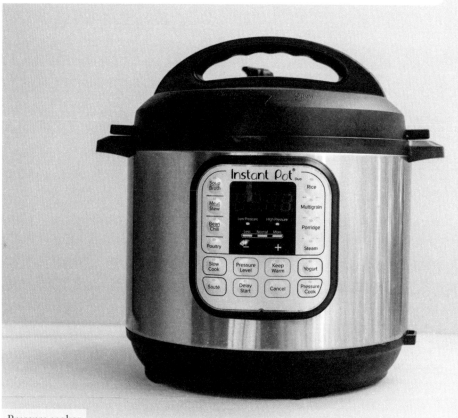

Pressure cooker

Straining infused oils

After straining your oil, placing it in a jar and labelling it, you might find that after a few days your lovely finished oil has accumulated sediment on the bottom of the jar or there are water droplets there. This is a normal process, and I like to take my oils that one step further to help preserve them and make them as pure as possible. There are a couple of methods here.

METHOD 1

As the water and sediment are likely to be on the bottom of the jar, I gently decant the top oil into another jar, making sure not to disturb the bottom. You will lose a small amount of the oil, but you will have a better oil without the potential mould-creating issues.

METHOD 2

This generally works best if you have Mason jars with wide lids – the ones that are as wide as the jar itself.

- *Make sure the lid is on as tight as possible to ensure there are no oil leakages.*

- *Stand the Mason jar on its lid so it is upside down. Let the sediment and water then float down to settle in the lid.*

- *Stick it lid down in the freezer for a few days. Oil takes a while to freeze!*

- *Take it out once it is really frozen and take the lid off. You should now be able to carefully scrape the impurities off the top, leaving the good oil underneath.*

TIPS:

- *Ensure no plant matter is sticking out above the oil. If it is, you run the risk of mould growing and you will have to throw your oil out.*

- *Store your oil in a jar that is close to full. The less air you have in the jar the better, as oils exposed to air will go rancid over time.*

- *Olive, sweet almond and sesame oils are the more stable oils. They will generally last longer before turning rancid.*

Preserving oils

Preserving your oils is a must if you don't intend to use them straight away. There is nothing worse than putting in great effort and using your sacred plant only for it to go rancid and end up unusable. To prevent your oil from going rancid you need to use an antioxidant – remember not to be confused with a preservative, which is different. Preservatives are used when there is water present in your product. For now you will need to add vitamin E, rosemary CO_2 extract or grapefruit seed extract to your oil. These are quite easy to find and relatively cheap. You only need to add 1% into your mix. They are generally added when the oil has cooled down. Rosemary CO_2 extract has quite a strong smell, so I generally use vitamin E. Wherever I state 'add vitamin E', you can interchange with the other options.

Weigh your finished oil and then add 1% vitamin E to the oil. To work this out, just simply multiply the amount you have i.e. 60 ml x 1%, which equals .6 ml.

NOTE: *do not add vitamin E if you are intending to ingest your oil.*

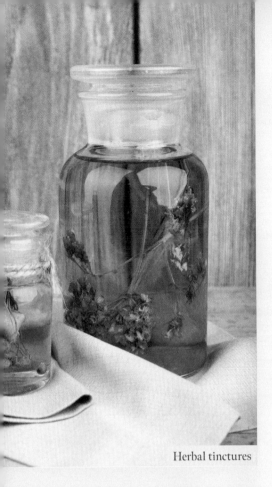

Herbal tinctures

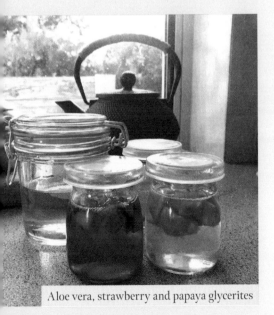

Aloe vera, strawberry and papaya glycerites

Glycerites/glycetracts

Glycerites – or glycetracts, as they are also known – are becoming increasingly popular among the home skincare community. They are great fun to make as well because you can practically use anything, even strawberries or cucumber! The solvent used in this case is glycerine – a thick, sweet-tasting and colourless liquid. Herbalists have used glycerites with great success for children or people who cannot tolerate alcohol tinctures. They not only taste nice, some don't require preserving because glycerine itself acts as a preservative. Ensure you get organic vegetable glycerine if you are going to ingest it. *If you add a preservative to your glycerite, do not ingest it.*

Glycerites retain the flavour, smell and colour of whatever you put in them, which makes them popular for colouring or flavouring products. My strawberry and cucumber ones smell amazing!

Glycerine works well for fresh plant extractions but is not so good for dry herbs, though it's doable providing you add water. The great thing about glycerites is that they can also be added to food. This is an excellent choice if you are undertaking a 'plant diet', which is a simple method of working with plant spirits. This involves ingesting the plant each day for a specified amount of time to gain a closer relationship to it. You might want to be creative and make specific cookies or muffins using your glycerite and place the flowers of the plant on the top, or maybe make a cooling drink with a herbal glycerite to honour the plant.

There are many recipes pertaining to cold and cough syrups using glycerine. Herbs like elderberry, licorice, thyme or marshmallow are often used. Herbs that are particularly mucilaginous – that is, producing a mucus-like gelatinous substance known as mucilage – such as marshmallow are enhanced with glycerine.

Flowers are great to use with glycerites and are used frequently to give products a beautiful colour, as the colour of the plant matter will colour the glycerine. You might want to use the flowers to colour your product and the other parts of the plant for either the water or oil part to make a cream, for instance, therefore using the entire plant. Once you start getting the hang of all the different ways you can extract properties, you can get highly creative!

Making glycerites is still largely experimental when it comes to using fresh plants or food

Glycerine also has a couple of different points to be aware of when used in making skincare products. When we make creams, the percentage of glycerine needed is only around 5–10% of the entire formula. At this percentage, glycerine draws moisture to the skin and is called a humectant. If the percentage is greater than 15% of your product formula the glycerine will start to draw moisture from the skin and can then sometimes irritate it due to dryness.

Glycerine has about 5% water content in it already, and we normally use 55–60% glycerine when making a glycetract, so glycerine makes up the majority of the jar. If you are using dried herbs to make your glycerite, if the glycerine exceeds 55% you do not need to use a preservative.

Making glycerites is still largely experimental when it comes to using fresh plants or food since we don't know exactly how much water content is in a plant or food, therefore it is hard to determine your glycerine to water ratio. It all depends on what plant matter you use. Experiment as much as you can, and you will get the hang of it.

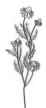

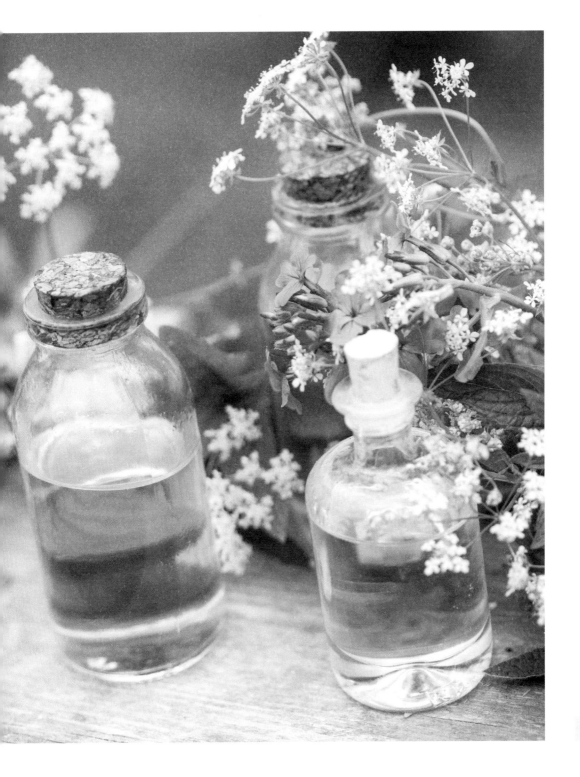

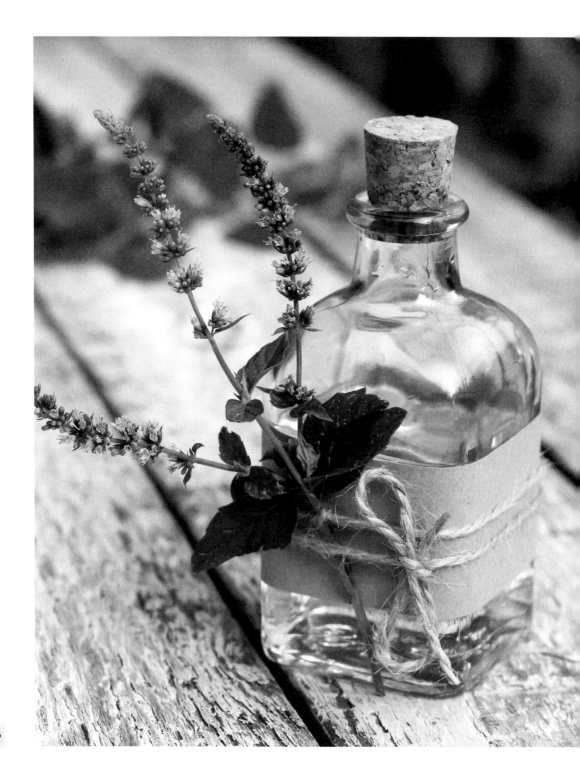

There are different methods depending on whether you are using dry or fresh herbs, as fresh herbs will always have water content in them. There are many methods for making glycerites, and I will share just a few in this book; it really comes down to experimenting. Don't be afraid to make mistakes. Just make everything in small batches to start with so you don't waste too much product. Considering glycerine is normally used at low percentages in products, a small amount will go a long way.

Now you might see in different places that glycerites should take anywhere from five days to six weeks to make. I just stick with 14 days but go with what feels right for you. Some may indeed take longer.

METHOD 1A: FRESH PLANT METHOD

You can use glycerine on its own for fresh plant matter because of the water content the glycerine will pull out. You can use fresh fruit, vegetables and flowers like strawberries, papaya, cucumber, aloe vera and hibiscus flowers, which seem to be popular, but the choices are endless. One simple method for making fresh fruit or vegetable glycetracts is as follows:

- *Chop up your matter and place it in your jar, filling it to about halfway.*

- *Fill the jar with glycerine.*

- *Shake daily for 14 days. You will notice your fruit or vegetables getting smaller as the water content is drained out of them into the glycerine.*

- *Strain through muslin cloth, jar and label.*

- *Add a preservative if required.*

I like to keep my glycerites in the fridge. You can add a preservative, but keep in mind your preservative will generally have a slight smell to it. This can overpower your glycerites at times.

METHOD 1B: DRIED PLANT METHOD

The dried plant method is the more accurate method because, as already explained, with fresh plant matter you cannot calculate exactly how much water is in the fresh plant, therefore you will never know what percentage of glycerine to water your glycerite makes. This leaves room for mould to grow if there is too much water, hence I sometimes add a preservative just in case.

As you can imagine, because glycerine is a thick substance it doesn't extract from dry substances well, so we need to add a little water to the mix to rehydrate the dry plant, which also helps extract its constituents.

- *Generally, to be safe, mix 70% glycerine with 30% water. (Other sources may say 60% glycerine.) Make your mix before pouring it over your herb. First, fill your jar with water to about ¾ full to calculate how much liquid in total you need. So if your jar takes 80 g/ml, multiply 80 by .7 (70%) to calculate the glycerine content, which equals 56 g/ml, and then subtract 56 from 80 to give you your water content: 24 g/ml (30%).*

- *Alternatively, you can make a mix using vinegar, which is another great solvent. Here you would use 30% glycerine, 30% vinegar and 40% water.*

- *You could add alcohol as another mix to a) help with the extraction process and b) act as a preservative. I would use 96% ethanol here at 10%, 30% water and 70% glycerine.*

- *Chop up your matter and place it in your jar, filling it to about halfway, keeping in mind that the dried plant will swell.*

- *Fill the jar with the glycerine mix you have created.*

- *Shake daily for 14 days.*

- *Strain through muslin cloth, jar and label.*

- *This shouldn't need a preservative as it has over 55% glycerine.*

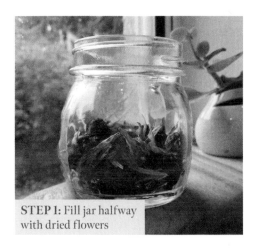

STEP 1: Fill jar halfway with dried flowers

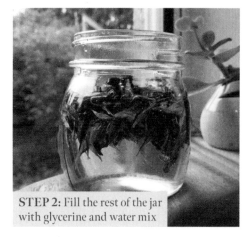

STEP 2: Fill the rest of the jar with glycerine and water mix

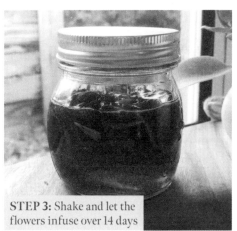

STEP 3: Shake and let the flowers infuse over 14 days

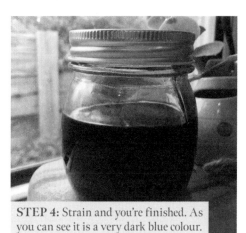

STEP 4: Strain and you're finished. As you can see it is a very dark blue colour.

METHOD 2: GLYCERITE BY REPLACEMENT

This is a handy method using an already created fluid extract/tincture. It's as simple as boiling off the alcohol and water and replacing it with glycerine.

- *Reduce your tincture in a water bath with the lid off to half its volume. The temperature needed to evaporate them is around 100°C/210°F.*

- *Add enough glycerine into the half mix to bring it up to its original volume. This will still be the same strength tincture, but now it is a glycerite.*

Infusion times

You will find different information on infusion times for glycerites. Just make it easy and stick to shaking it twice a day for 14 days.

Oxymels/syrups

Oxymels or syrups are another fun way of extracting plant properties. They not only taste good, but they are also very soothing on your throat and digestive system. Elderberry syrup is a common one. It's a wonderful way to ingest your plant because it's so versatile. You can drizzle them on your food (they make awesome salad dressings), add them to your drinks or even drink a teaspoon of them neat. They do, however, contain a lot of sugar in the form of honey, so keep this in mind. Everything in moderation is the key message.

Vinegar is a solvent that can help extract the properties of the herbs, and honey is then added to give it a nice taste and also act as a preservative. Using dry herbs is best so the water content can't dilute the vinegar and give something for mould and bacteria to grow in. However, fresh garlic is an exception and is widely beneficial on many levels when added if you can stomach the taste. These kinds of mixes were used hundreds of years ago, as vinegar, honey and dried herbs were easy to acquire. They are fun and easy to make, and most are relatively nice to the taste. Rose-scented geranium is a favourite of mine for making into a syrup.

Again, there are a few methods for making oxymels and syrups. Essentially, you either make a vinegar infusion with your plant matter and then add honey, or you can add the vinegar and honey to the plant matter first and let it sit for a few weeks to months. The method is the same as with infusing oils, just with vinegar instead. Basically, we are going to do a 1:1 mix – i.e. one part vinegar and one part honey. You might see different ratios in different books. There is no right or wrong, so start with one part each until you get the hang of it. If you are not a fan of the vinegar taste, change the ratio to more honey.

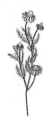

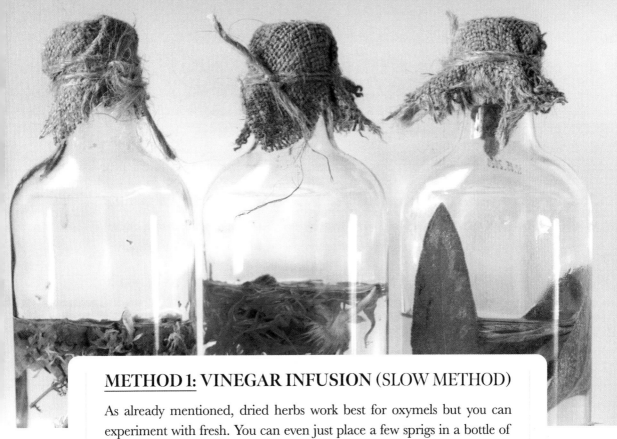

METHOD 1: VINEGAR INFUSION (SLOW METHOD)

As already mentioned, dried herbs work best for oxymels but you can experiment with fresh. You can even just place a few sprigs in a bottle of vinegar to impart the flavour and make a beautiful gift.

- *Grind or finely chop your dried plant matter.*

- *It is up to you how much herb/plant you want to use. I generally fill a jar to ⅓ full. The plant matter will expand in the jar. Weigh your plant matter first and write down how much it weighs in your notebook.*

- *Place your plant matter into your jar. Use a jar with a plastic lid for vinegars, as they can corrode your metal lids.*

- *Pour your vinegar into a measuring jug so you can measure how much you are going to put in the jar and how much is needed to cover the plant.*

- *Cover the plant matter with vinegar and add a little more to allow for the plant matter to expand, then record how much vinegar you used.*

- *Let it sit for 10 to 14 days, shaking every day.*

- *Strain and weigh your final amount.*

- *If you wish to keep your vinegar as it is, you will need to heat it close to boiling point and then filter it while it is hot. This process helps prolong the life of your vinegar by delaying rapid fermentation.*

- *If you continue to make the oxymel, heat the vinegar close to a boil in a water bath and add the same amount of honey to your vinegar i.e. if you have 150 ml of vinegar add the same amount of honey. Keep it on the heat and simmer it until it turns to the consistency of syrup.*

- **Note** – *the mix will still look liquid as it is reducing. Take a little tester out with a spoon, let it cool down and taste it to see how you like it. Having it in the Pyrex jug also allows you to monitor how much it has reduced i.e. if you have 300 ml total volume in the jug – if you reduce it by half, wait until it gets down to 150 ml and then it's done.*

- *Bottle and label.*

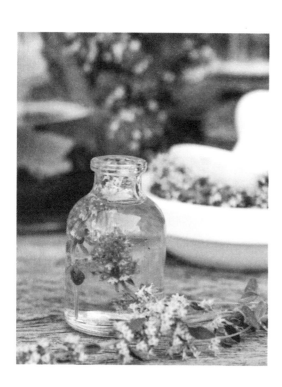

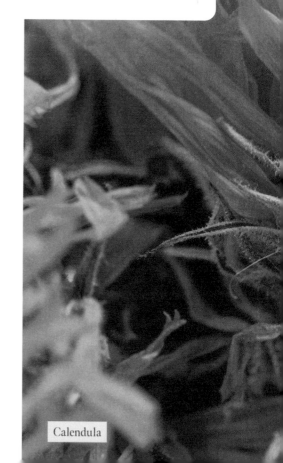

Calendula

METHOD 2: VINEGAR AND HONEY INFUSION (SLOW METHOD)

- *Grind or finely chop your dried plant matter.*

- *Weigh your plant matter, and write down how much it weighs in your notebook.*

- *Place your plant matter into your jar to about ⅓ full. Use a jar with a plastic lid for vinegars, as they can corrode metal lids.*

- *Add both the honey and vinegar to nearly fill the jar. Mix it first in a jug before pouring over your plant matter. You might want to find out how much liquid your jar holds first by pouring some vinegar into it to nearly full and then pouring it into a measuring jug. Divide that amount by two and that will give roughly the quantity you need of vinegar and honey.*

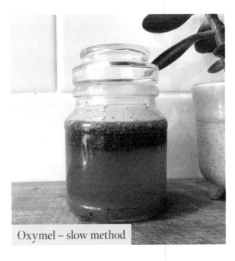

Oxymel – slow method

- *Let it sit for 10 to 14 days, shaking it every day.*

- *Strain, bottle and label or heat the mix up in a water bath and reduce to a syrup.*

METHOD 3: HEATED VINEGAR INFUSION (FAST METHOD)

We don't always have time to wait up to 14 days for our vinegar infusions, so there is another, faster method that works equally as well. Heating the herbs in vinegar, just like doing our heated oils, is the fast method. It takes about 20 minutes to make the vinegar infusion and then you can decide whether you want to reduce it down to a syrup.

RECIPE: ROSE-SCENTED GERANIUM OXYMEL SYRUP

Here is a quick recipe I love to make out of my dried rose-scented geraniums. Start with a small batch to see how you like it. If you don't want to reduce it down to a syrup, it tastes amazing as just an oxymel. It makes a beautiful salad dressing! You can make it with either fresh or dried leaves.

Rose-scented geranium is used in skincare to balance out the skin. It also works on the nervous system, relieves stress, helps calm anxiety and may be of benefit for depression. On a spiritual level, it has traditionally been used to protect against negative energy. It also helps with balance and uplifts your vibration.

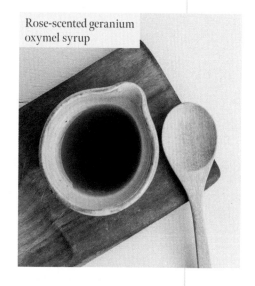

Rose-scented geranium oxymel syrup

I'm using millilitres in this recipe mainly because I am using a Pyrex jug to measure a 1:1 ratio of vinegar to honey. It also helps to see when you have reduced it down by half because you can easily measure it on the side of the jug. The amount of herb will obviously depend on if you use fresh or dried herb and how finely you have cut it down. If you weigh everything as you go and write it down you can easily convert those amounts to percentages, which I explain in detail in the next chapter.

- *Grind or finely chop your dried leaves.*

- *Place 50 ml of apple cider vinegar in a Pyrex jug and then add your herb to it, enough so that the vinegar is full of herb and still liquid enough for the herb to float around in it.*

- *Place in a water bath and bring the water in the bath to a simmer. Simmer the mix for 15 minutes.*

- *Strain the mix – I use a coffee filter over another Pyrex jug. You will need to squeeze the mix to get all the liquid out. You should still have around 50 ml of vinegar. Add 50 ml of honey so it reads 100 ml on the jug.*

- *Place it back in the water bath and simmer until it reduces to a syrup. I reduce mine by half, so it should reduce back down to around 50 ml, which can take around an hour or so. It may still look watery, so do a taste test. You will notice it feels thicker when you taste it. Remember to check on it from time to time while it is on the stove, as the water in the bath also evaporates. Add more boiling water from a jug to it if necessary.*

- *Once it has reached a good consistency, let it cool completely before pouring it into a bottle or you will get condensation in the bottle, which can create mould and bacteria. Label as appropriate.*

Succi

Succi is the name given to the juice you obtain by pulping fresh plant material. This needs to be used straight away as it can be hard to preserve. It could be applied neat to the skin in some instances, such as chickweed or comfrey, for example. If needed for longer than 24 hours, you would need to preserve it with around 30% ethanol, let it sit for about 14 days and then filter it. It might then last six months.

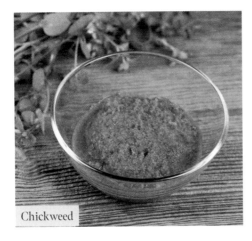

Chickweed

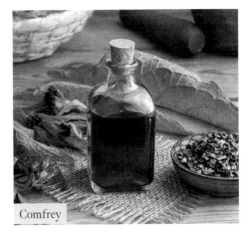

Comfrey

Plant essences

Plant essences are similar to homeopathic remedies, where the water itself contains the vibrational essence of the plant, just like Bach Flower Remedies or Australian Bush Flower Essences. They are made in the same way as the flower essences. They are convenient to travel with, safe for pets, plants and children and perfect to include in room sprays.

Generally you take about seven drops of the essence under your tongue morning and night, but if you have made up something to take like an emergency essence you would take it whenever you feel you need it. Plant essences won't interact with any medications you are taking, and you can't overdose on them. However, everything in moderation.

Equipment

The first thing you need to think about is do you need to create a single dose bottle to last a week or do you want it to last longer, which requires an alcohol to preserve it? Brandy, vodka or gin works best here. You don't need much, so buying the little miniatures can be a cost-effective solution if you are making only a couple.

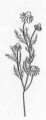

You will also need:

- **A vessel to contain the water,** remembering a dose is only seven drops each time so you don't need a huge bowl. Depending on how much you want to make, you could pick a small glass jar or a large glass jug. You can even use a small glass jar to house the plant matter in and place that inside a larger glass jar or jug that you fill with water. This way the plant is essentially inside the water vessel but not touching the water. This is perfect if the plant is toxic in any way.

- **A small 30 ml amber dropper bottle** and a glass jar to contain your essence once made.

- **Good clean water.** What water should you use? It's important to use as pure a water as you can. Filtered tap water or bottled water from glass bottles is ok. Take care with any plastic bottled water – take into consideration the impact on the environment, where it is water mined from and the chemical leaching from the plastic into the bottle. Do your best to source as pure as possible.

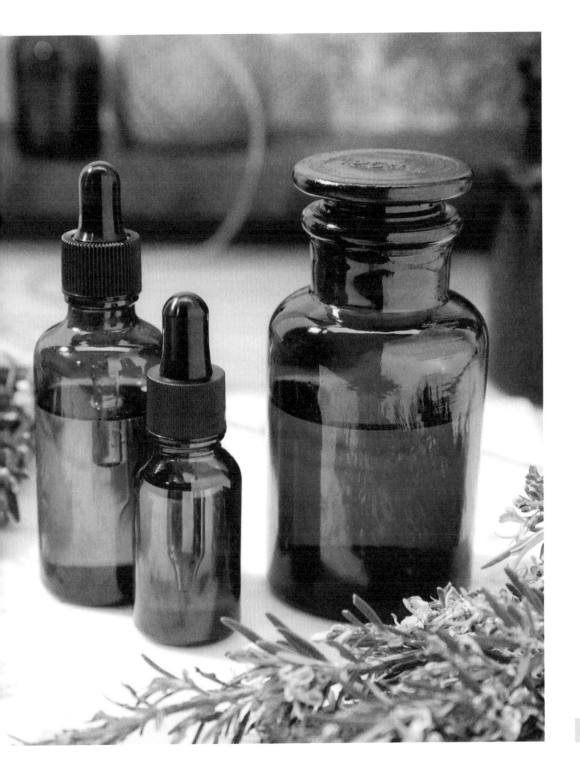

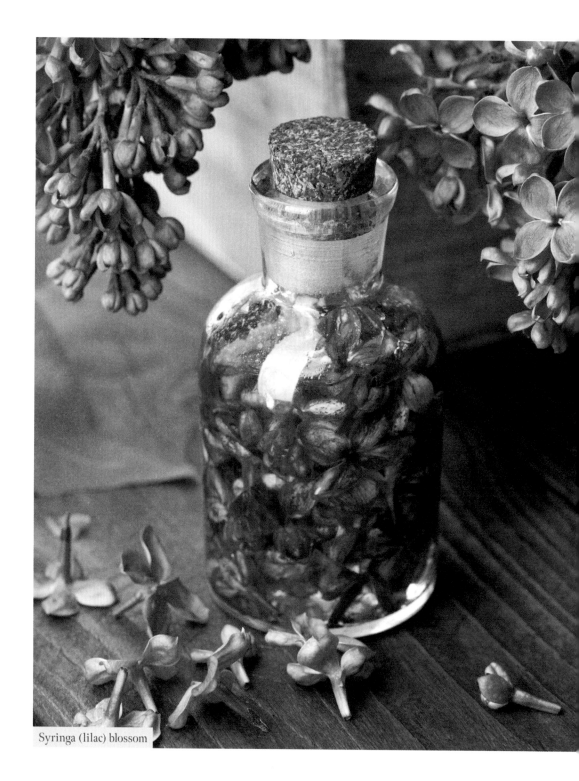

Syringa (lilac) blossom

Creation and preservation

Flower essences are generally made out in the sun for around four hours, so if you want to make yours outside the sun is a great way to help your plants infuse into the water – just make sure it's not going to get too hot. A little warmth is good. You can also use the moonlight – the full moon is great – and you can then leave overnight.

Firstly, have your vessel of water ready and sit with your plant to ask if you may pick some parts of it to place in water to create an essence for the benefit of healing. Then pick what feels right to place in the water. This might be when the flowers are at full peak and open, or you might use fresh new leaves. Use your intuition and let yourself be guided here.

How long you need to leave your essence in the sun will vary depending on the situation or the time you have available, so use your intuition here. If you know it will be disturbed at some stage, finish it before then. If the weather changes or you feel it's time to finish it, then do. If leaving outside overnight, you might like to drape something light over the water vessel to ensure dust and other things don't land in it.

Once it is finished, make sure you finish it all with the same focus and intent that you started with. Thank the plants for their help, strain and pour it into a bottle or jar.

You then want to preserve its life or make what's called a mother tincture: fill a small bottle halfway with alcohol and add your plant essence to fill up the other half. Thump the bottom of the bottle on the palm of your hand a couple of times to mix it. This is now your mother tincture bottle. From that bottle you would then add five to seven drops of mother tincture to a 30 ml dropper bottle filled with 50/50 alcohol and water. Give this another thump on your palm to mix again. This is now your stock bottle. From your stock bottle, you can create what's called your dosage bottles. The dosage bottle is what you use daily as your essence. Fill another bottle with 50/50 alcohol and water, and then put five to seven drops in the bottle and mix again – this is now your dosage bottle. From there you can take seven drops under your tongue when needed.

By making stock bottles you can create a dosage bottle made of many different flower essences. I generally don't exceed more than seven in a bottle. You would then put five to seven drops of each flower essence into the dosage bottle. Make sure you label to say what's in it!

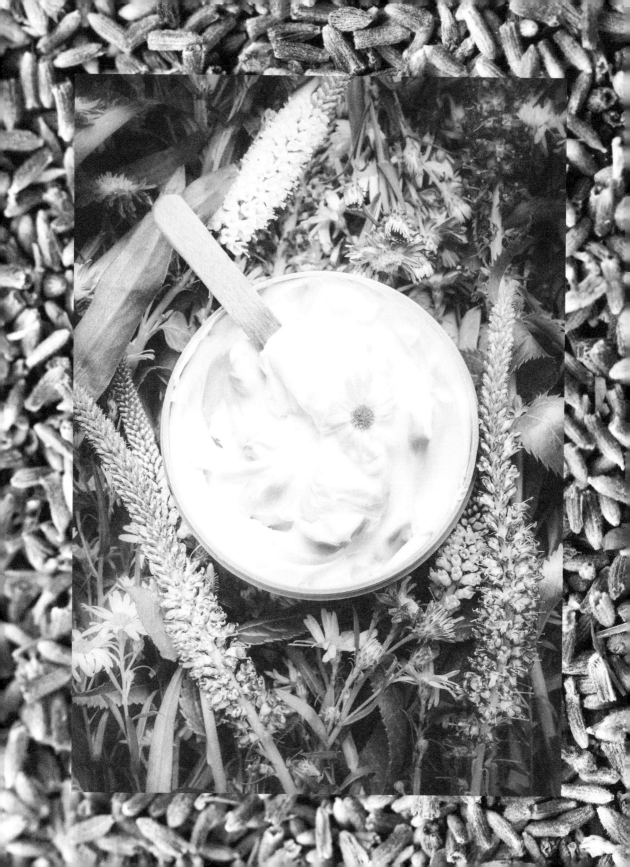

CHAPTER 6

Before you start making

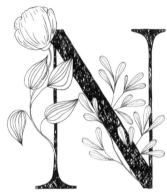

ow that we have our plant extraction, we need to decide what we want to make! If you have made a big batch of a herbal extract, there are so many things you can make. You need to think what's the most effective way to use it: in a salve, a cream, a room spray? Does it need to sit on the surface of the skin, which would require more of an ointment base? Is it for personal use, or will it be for others? Let your intuition guide you as well. Experiment, research, look for inspiration online. Be as creative as you like and try not to copy others. Of course, when you are starting out it's ok to do this to understand how to make things, but once you know what you are doing try to do something a bit different. I know it's easy to see something awesome someone else has made, but you really need to make it your own. Build on what you see in other products and also let spirit guide you.

But before we get into the heart of Plant Spirit Medicine making, first you need to know how to calculate the right amounts for your products and how to label correctly.

Calculations

When I first started making products, I never knew how to make the right amount of anything to fill just one jar. It wasn't until I had a product contract manufactured that I discovered they used percentages to calculate the ingredients instead of their measurements in millilitres or grams. Calculating by percentages means that if you have two 15 g jars that you want to make up you can calculate exactly what you need to fill them, so there is no wastage. Percentages are also great because it doesn't matter what country you are from and what measurement system you use, you can work it out in your preferred weight measurements.

You might want to mark this page on how to calculate percentages, as I'll be giving all my examples in them. Trust me, this will be so helpful! Once you get the hang of it all you'll be able to play with your ingredients and percentages, and it will make life easier for you in the long run. This will give you the ability to modify your recipes and make them your own.

First things first

Your formula should always equal 100%. Here is a basic formula for a cream:

Shea butter	50%
Oil	49%
Vitamin E (antioxidant)	1%
TOTAL	**100%**

The oil could be any infused oil you have made and can be any oil. Note that it also has an antioxidant to prevent the oils from going rancid.

Say I want to make a 15 g jar of this product. We always divide the percentage of each ingredient by 100 first, and then multiply it by the size of the jar you need to fill. Here is the equation:

Percentages to grams:
Percentage of ingredient divided by 100 multiplied by the total grams needed.
% ÷ 100 x total grams needed.

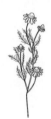

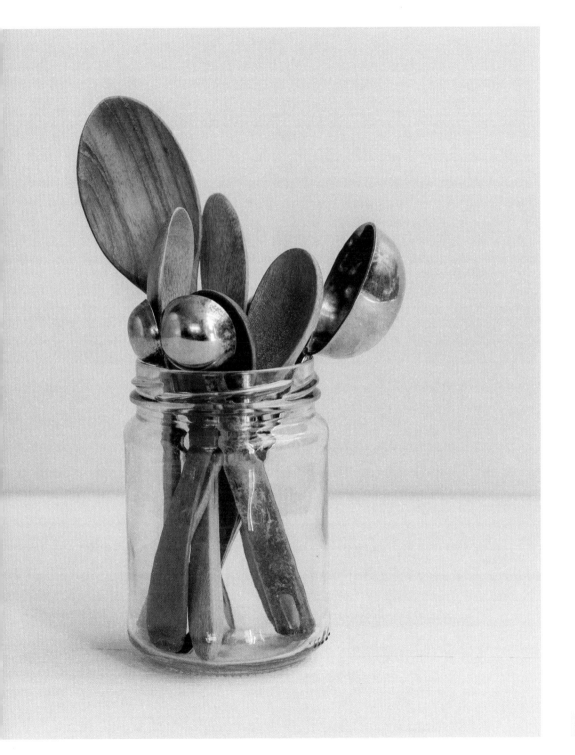

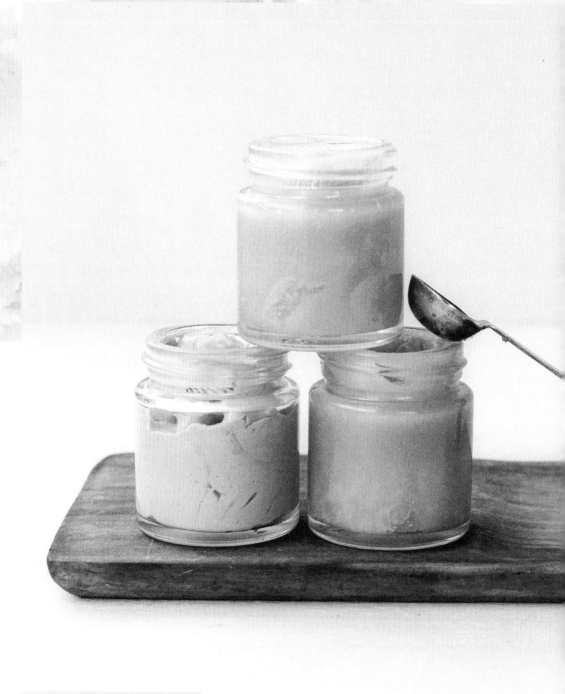

Hibiscus, hemp and comfrey creams

So if we want to make 15 g of this formula, it's calculated as follows:

Shea butter	50 divided by 100 multiplied by 15	=	7.5 g
Oil	49 divided by 100 multiplied by 15	=	7.35 g
Vitamin E (antioxidant)	1 divided by 100 multiplied by 15	=	0.15 g
	TOTAL	=	**15 g**

What if we have a bottle that takes liquid in millilitres?

Easy, we have to know how many ml the bottle takes. You might want to fill it up with a liquid to find out first, then use the above formula using ml instead of grams.

What if we know the grams of a formula but want to know the percentages?

Keep in mind the total percentage of any formula should add up to 100%. If you have a formula already in grams but with a random total, you can convert it to percentages using another easy sum:

Grams to percentages:

Number of grams per ingredient multiplied by 100, divided by the total numbers of grams in the formula.

Grams x 100 ÷ total grams in the formula.

For example, if we had a formula in grams and not percentages we would calculate it like this:

Shea butter	45 g
Oil	25 g
Vitamin E (antioxidant)	1 g
TOTAL	**71 g**

Shea butter	45 multiplied by 100 divided by 71	=	63.4
Sweet almond oil	25 multiplied by 100 divided by 71	=	35.2
Vitamin E (antioxidant)	1 multiplied by 100 divided by 71	=	1.4
		TOTAL	**=**	**100%**

You can round the numbers up or down to make it easier to measure out if needed.

Once you get your head around these two formulas it will make life easier when you need to make specific batch sizes. You can convert any formula to percentages if you know the weights, and from there you can then calculate what you need for any size or amount. If you have a recipe that is in tablespoons, grams and millilitres, just weigh each ingredient so you have everything in grams first. So if your recipe contains two tablespoons, weigh how much they are and weigh the millilitres so everything is in grams.

How to change a formula

Once you have your recipe converted into percentages, you can alter your recipe easily. All you need to remember is your recipe always needs to add up to 100%. Knowing this, if you need to add something to your formula, say an essential oil of .5%, you simply reduce something else in your formula, like the oil for example, down by .5%. Always keep your antioxidant or preservative in the formula the same at 1%. Keep your essential oils to a maximum of 1% when getting started, so if you are using more than one essential oil the total of the essential oils you put in should add up to 1%. You can go above 1% up to 5%, but some essential oils have a maximum percentage allowed so do the research on your specific essential oil.

> NOTE: *as a rule, no more than 1% essential oils should go into a formula that will go on the face, 0.5% for anything on the lips and 0.1% around the eyes. I prefer no essential oils for the eye area.*

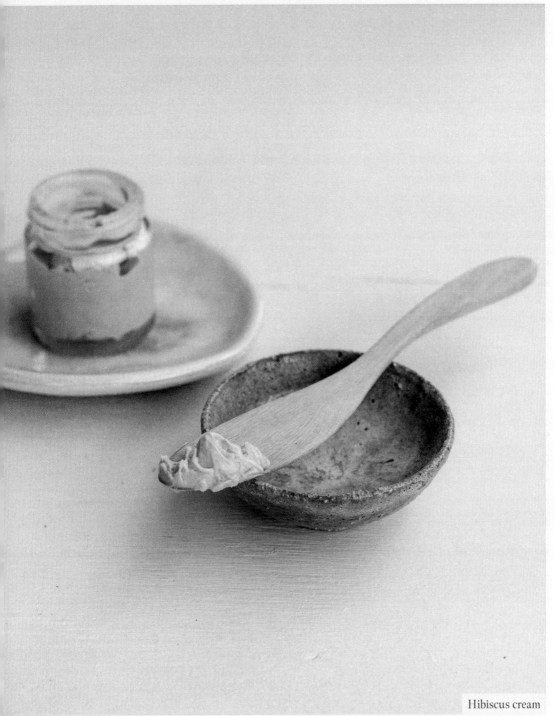

Hibiscus cream

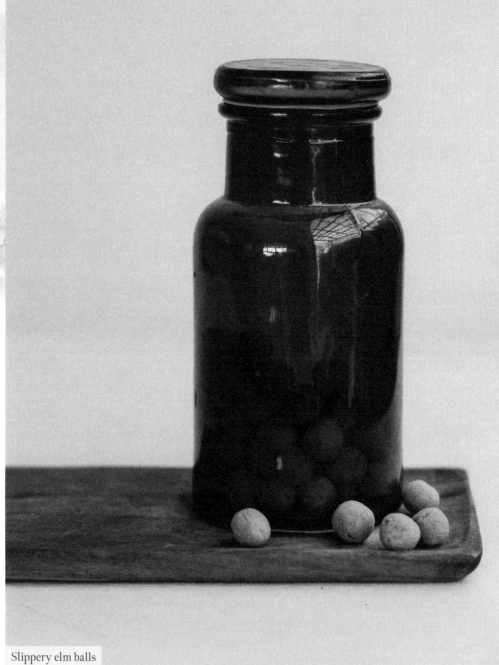

Slippery elm balls

This would be your new formula:

Shea butter	50%
Oil	48.5%
Vitamin E (antioxidant)	1%
Essential oil	0.5%
TOTAL	**100%**

Our infused oils and glycerites etc are very dear to us by the time we have made them, so you might not want to use much in each formula. A general rule is use up to 10% in your formula of your infused botanical.

I tend to use small percentages of my infused oils when it comes to making creams, but you can of course use all of your infused oil in a recipe. I use 100% in salves and ointments. If you choose to use 10%, if your recipe calls for 49% oil, you could use 39% oil and 10% of your infused oil.

Glycerites should always be used up to 10% only in any product, as glycerine in higher percentages can be drying to your skin.

How do I know what percentages to use?

There are some basic rules to help you create the right consistency when creating your products. For instance, for harder products you need wax and hard butters while for soft products you need more oils and water ingredients.

Now that we know how to use formulas with percentages, I urge you to experiment using small amounts of ingredients first. This is the great thing about percentages: you can make up tiny 20 g batches to check if your formula works before making a big batch and wasting your sacred ingredients by making a mistake. I purchase a whole lot of 25 g glass jars to put all my trials in and use tiny 40 ml beakers to mix everything up in. Plus, making little batches is quick.

Labelling

As already mentioned, labelling is extremely important – even more so now that we are making up products. People need to be able to read what's in a product to determine if there is something in there that they are allergic to. The label should also tell them how to use it and who to contact should they have a reaction or need to buy more. It is hard to put an expiry date on home-made products, and it really depends on what kind of product it is and what you have put in it.

Because we are not making therapeutic products, your product may be classed as a cosmetic. Depending on which country you live in, you may legally need to put what's called the 'INCI' names of your ingredients on your label – INCI stands for International Nomenclature of Cosmetic Ingredients. This is the Latin or botanical name as discussed earlier, e.g. *Calendula officinalis* is calendula. This helps create a uniform way of declaring what is in your product, so people can quickly determine exactly what has been used no matter where in the world you live. However, it does confuse the consumer unless they understand these names, so I like to include both.

Here is an example of how you might label an oil

If you have used an infused oil of calendula with almond oil and your oil is your main ingredient, it would be the first to appear in your ingredient list and may read:

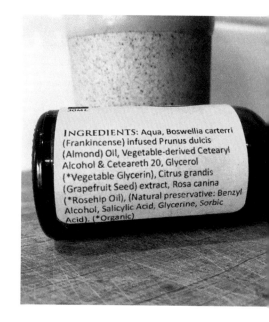

> *Calendula officinalis* (calendula) infused *Prunus dulcus* (almond) oil.

> OR *Calendula officinalis* infused *Prunus dulcus* oil.

> OR calendula-infused almond oil (if your country does not require the INCI name).

Details every label should contain:

- **What's in your bottle** – list every ingredient, whether herb, water, alcohol etc., in descending order according to how much is in the product. So if you use 70% almond oil, 20% butter and 10% of other ingredients, you list from highest to lowest.

- **Dosage/directions** – it's important to explain how much to use so people don't go overboard. Tell them exactly how and where to use it. Don't assume people will just know.

- **Date created** – this helps you know when you made something; it helps the owner of the product decide when something should not be used; and it may also help you if someone has a reaction to your product, so you can work back to see what you used and where you got it from.

- **Name of recipient if needed**

- **Contact details**

- **Essential oil sensitisers** – in some countries, like in the EU, you need to list what's called sensitisers on your label. Specific essential oils like geranium, for example, have substances in them that are known allergens for some people. These essential oils have specific dermal limits, meaning they should not exceed certain percentages in your formulations. This is why it is critical to research each and every essential oil you add to your formula. The sensitiser for geranium is geraniol, and you would need to ensure that you have the safe amount in your formula and place its name on your label.

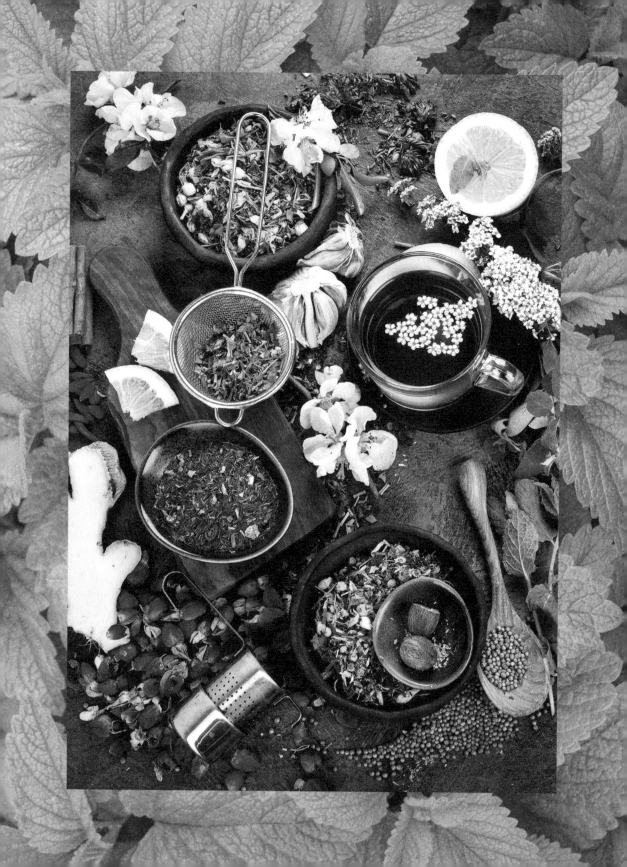

CHAPTER 7

Plant Spirit Medicine making

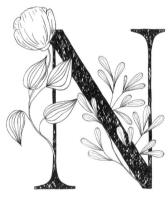

Now that we have covered how to extract your plant material, how to calculate your ingredients and how to label your products, it's time to think about what you can now make. The options really are endless here. You can use your oils on their own, you can create massage or bath oils, or you can use them in salves, balms, ointments, lotions and creams. If you have created them with edible plants and oils like olive oil, macadamia nut, avocado oil etc. you can use them in your cooking, over vegies, as dressings etc. You might even like to make fragrant oils that you put in roll-on bottles like a perfume, so you can smell the scent of your plant all day long. Essential oils can be added to your oils, again keeping to around 1%. If you are an aromatherapist you will know which oils you can increase. I suggest you do further reading or research on aromatherapy if this interests you. This book does not cover the topic as it is too extensive.

As with any oil, you will need to add an antioxidant to keep it from going rancid. If you have created an oil for eating, do not add vitamin E at any stage. If you are making a massage oil, anointing oil or any other type of oil, all you need do is mix whatever oils you like together and add 1% vitamin E and up to 1% of essential oils if required. If all your oils already have vitamin E in them from the infusing process, there should be no need to add any extra.

Salves and balms

Salves and balms are easily the most popular product to make. Not only are they simple to make, they have so many uses and are great to take on your travels. Another great thing about them is they only need an antioxidant to keep them stable because they contain no water.

Basically all we do with salves and balms is heat our infused oil up in a water bath and add beeswax or plant wax to the oil. When cooling, add some vitamin E and pour into jars. You can add essential oils at this stage also.

If you are making a vegan product, you might like to use candelilla wax – a natural plant wax that works just as well as beeswax. A 1:5 ratio of wax to oil using candelilla works for me, but again there is no hard and fast rule. Many people use a 1:4 ratio using

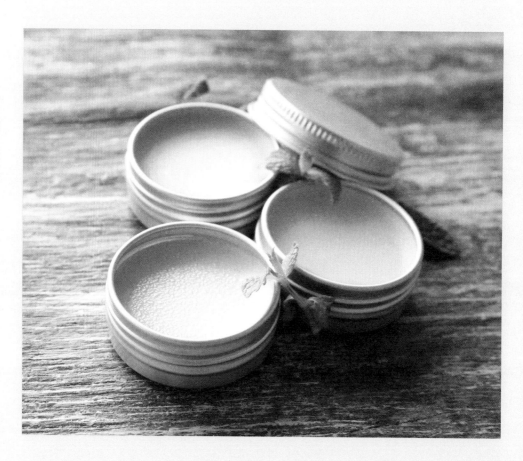

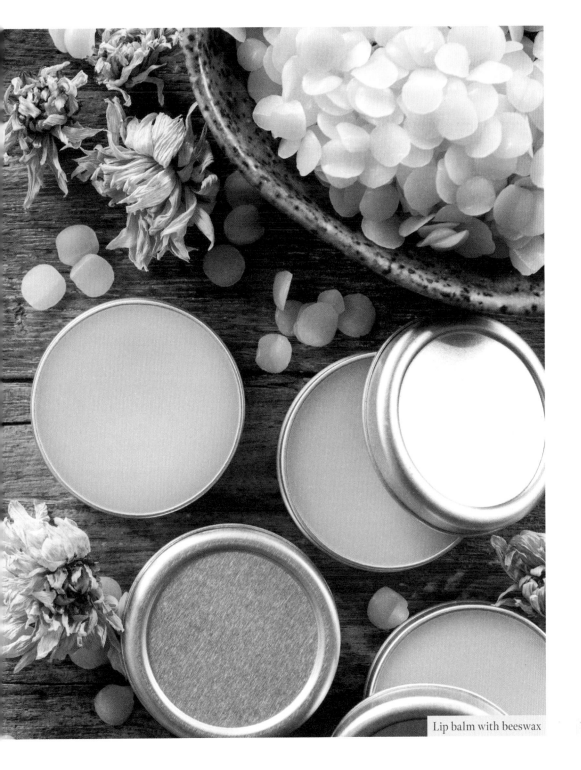

Lip balm with beeswax

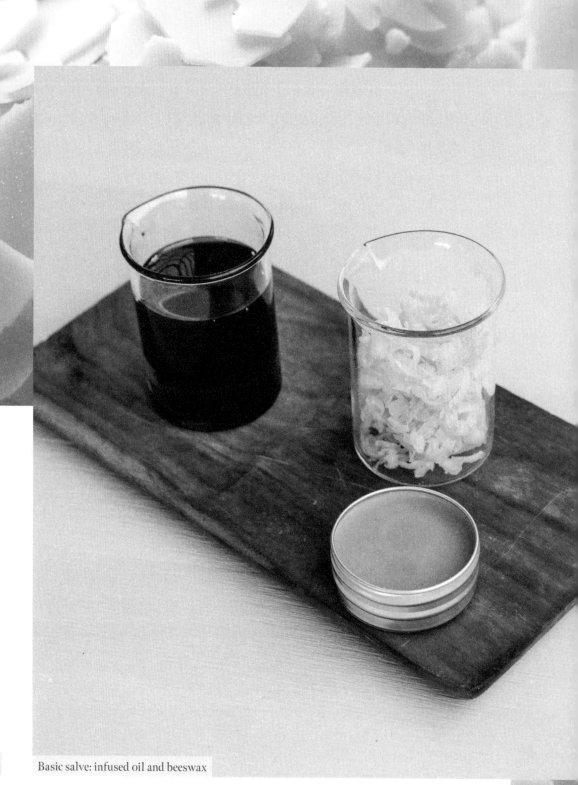

Basic salve: infused oil and beeswax

beeswax and sometimes it will differ depending on what type of oil you use. To find what works for you, when you have your oil and wax heating on the stove and the wax has completely dissolved, take a little amount out and drop one drop onto something cold. It will solidify quickly, and you will get an indication of what it will be like when it cools. If it is too liquid, simply add more wax; if it is too hard, add more oil.

RECIPE: BASIC SALVE/BALM

For a basic salve or balm, I use a 1:5 mix of wax to oil. So if I need 30 g of salve, which is enough to fill two 15 g jars (a standard lip balm jar), I would use 5 g of wax and 25 g of oil. With ratios you add the numbers together, in this case 1 + 5 = 6. Then divide the finished quantity you need by that number, in our case it is 30 g divided by 6 = 5 g. We then know that one part equals 5 g and the 5 parts needed is 5 x 5 = 25 g.

Vitamin E will make up part of that 25 g and we know it needs to be 1% of the formulation. If the total weight is 30 g and we need to know how much 1% of that is, we multiply 30 by .01 or 30 multiplied by 1%, which makes it 0.3 g. We then take the 0.3 g off the 25 g of oil to leave 24.7 g of oil needed, making it 24.7 g of infused oil, with 0.3 g of vitamin E, as per below.

Here is where we will use the grams to percentages calculation from the previous chapter to determine our percentages. Always make your formulas show both. Here is the calculation:

Grams x 100 ÷ total grams of the formula.

Which equals:

24.7 g x 100 ÷ 30 g = 82.3%
5 g x 100 ÷ 30 g = 16.7%
0.3 g x 100 ÷ 30 g = 1%

Feel free to round the percentages to the closest number if needed, i.e. 82.3% = 82%, 16.7% = 17% and vitamin E 1%. Just always ensure your totals add up to 100%.

Infused oil	82.3%	=	24.7g
Candelilla/beeswax	16.7%	=	5 g
Vitamin E	1%	=	0.3 g
TOTAL	**100%**	**=**	**30 g**

Alternatively, if you want to add an essential oil you could use the recipe as follows:

Infused oil	81.3%	=	24.4 g
Candelilla/beeswax	16.7%	=	5 g
Essential oil	1%	=	0.3 g
Vitamin E	1%	=	0.3 g
TOTAL	**100%**	**=**	**30 g**

METHOD:

- *Heat up the oil and wax together in a water bath until the wax melts completely. Take off the stove and let cool down a little. Vitamin E and essential oils are heat sensitive, so you have to add them in the cooling down phase. I find this a bit tricky because as it cools it hardens, and you need to pour the mix into jars before it sets. It can be a bit of a balancing act. If the mix starts to harden in your pouring jug, place it quickly back into the water bath to help it melt again and pour it into jars as quick as you can.*

- *Always leave the lid off the jar until the product has completely cooled down. If it is still warm, condensation can cause mould to grow in the jar.*

Lavender balms are a good one to make – I make them from my own lavender-infused oil and lavender essential oil. They smell amazing and are great to help you relax and find calm, but are also great for burns, cuts and scrapes. Lavender is one of those terrific all-rounders.

I started off my Plant Spirit Medicine making with palo santo balms, which were absolutely amazing. I made them by infusing the sawdust in oil. This allowed me to use less palo santo than you would normally use for smudging with sticks. You can use the balm and call on the spirit of the palo santo tree when you use it. You can anoint your tools and yourself. However, due to the sustainability issues of the tree, I needed

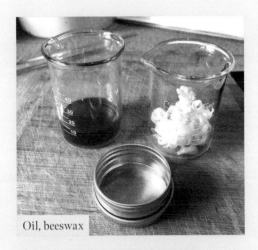

Oil, beeswax

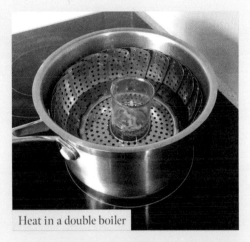

Heat in a double boiler

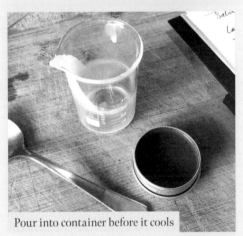

Pour into container before it cools

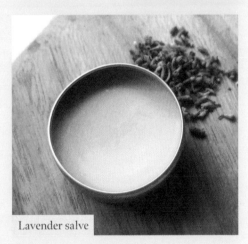

Lavender salve

to cease promoting it. This may change over time if the situation alters, who knows, but for now it just doesn't feel right.

I also make a vervain balm and mugwort balm. I am also now growing my own herbs to make into salves, like white sage. Once you start you get hooked!

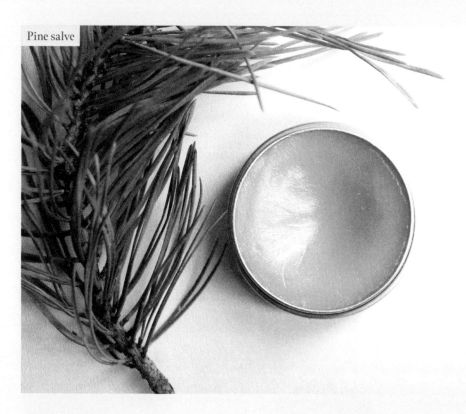

Pine salve

Ointments

Ointments are oil-based preparations and are designed to stay on the surface of the skin to help deliver the herbal ingredients to it. They are generally used for skin conditions like eczema, cuts and wounds. Because they stay on the surface of the skin, they are quite greasy. Infused oils and resins work great in ointments, but you can also add a small amount of tincture to them or powdered herbs. Anhydrous lanolin can absorb up to half its weight in liquid. Lanolin has a strong smell though, so it's good to keep this ingredient low unless you have some strong essential oils to mask the smell.

I've created a great recipe for an ointment base that is similar to petroleum jelly. You can add powders and essential oils to it, and it spreads really well. Bear in mind, it does sit on the surface of the skin due to its oil content. As you can see by the formula, it contains 60% oil. You can add your infused oil as the main oil or break it down a bit, by adding say 20% of your infused oil and 40% olive oil. It all depends on what your intentions are for the ointment. Being a Plant Spirit Medicine, I like these blends because they sit on your skin and you can keep smelling them.

As mentioned earlier, lanolin can also act as an emulsifier in that it can hold up to half its weight in water. So if you want to incorporate a tincture into the mix add it while the mix is melted over heat, and obviously you would need to adjust the percentages so it adds up to 100%. If you were to add say 5% herbal tincture, you might adjust the amount of oil you have by 5%.

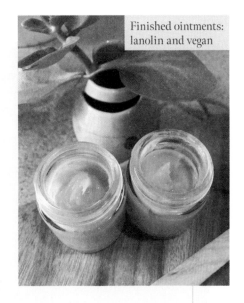

Finished ointments: lanolin and vegan

RECIPE: BASIC OINTMENT

Olive oil	60%
Lanolin	20%
Beeswax	19%
Vitamin E	1%
TOTAL	**100%**

METHOD:

- *Place all ingredients, except the vitamin E, in a glass jar or beaker and place in a double boiler/water bath until everything has melted.*

- *Remove from the heat and let cool, but keep stirring. As it is starting to set, add the vitamin E and essential oils if required and stir in well.*

- *Pour into jars before it sets. If it sets before getting in the jars, return to the heat quickly to remelt. This can be a bit of a balancing act, but you'll soon get the hang of it. Remember, also, vitamin E and essential oils are heat sensitive and reheating can be damaging, so be quick if you absolutely have to.*

- *Once set, I like to give it a big stir. Just gouge a spoon or knife in and mix it as much as you can. This gives it a creamy consistency, and then it's ready to either use on its own (if you have used an infused oil in it) or you can add essential oils and powders. Measure out a small amount before putting them in, so you will know how much the mix can take and you can replicate it again.*

I create a big batch of it to keep as a base product. Then when I need some I scoop out a small jar full, add my powdered herbs to it and I'm done! You can also add a few drops of essential oils to it – just ensure you mix it well.

Remember lanolin has a strong odour, so if you want to add essential oils for their aroma you might want to reduce the lanolin to 10% and perhaps increase your oil and wax by 5% each. Play around until you get the consistency that works for you.

For a vegan alternative you could use the following, but it won't get the same consistency without lanolin. However, I'm sure you could find a butter or maybe a resin to add to it that might help. Maybe pine resin, as it is an oil-soluble and soft resin, or you could add some soy lecithin.

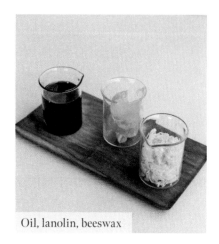
Oil, lanolin, beeswax

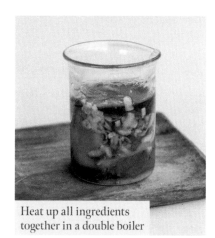
Heat up all ingredients together in a double boiler

Lanolin has a strong odour, so if you want to add essential oils for their aroma … reduce the lanolin to 10%

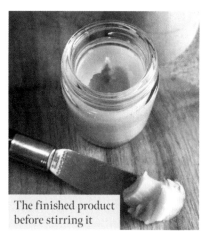
The finished product before stirring it

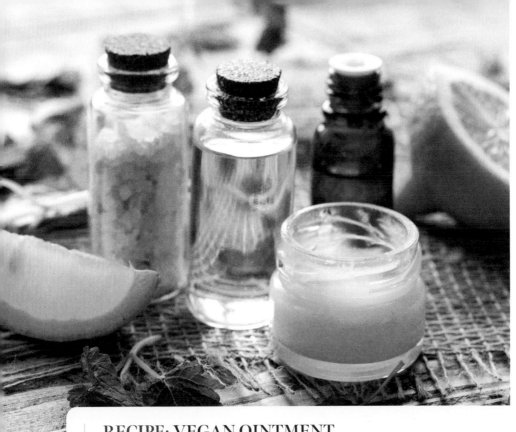

RECIPE: VEGAN OINTMENT

Olive oil	80%
Candelilla wax	19%
Vitamin E	1%
TOTAL	**100%**

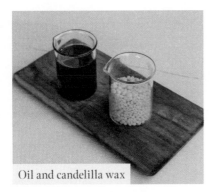

Oil and candelilla wax

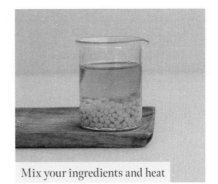

Mix your ingredients and heat

Another oil you might look at using here would be castor oil.

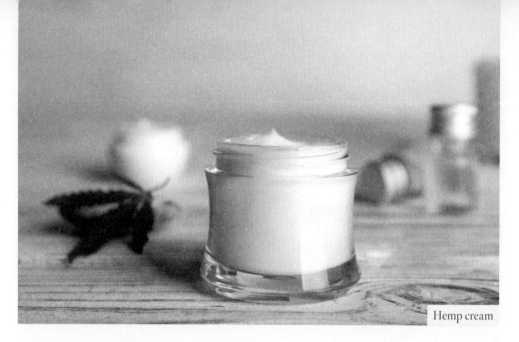

Hemp cream

Lotions/creams

Creams and lotions are the first group of water-based products that we are going to make, which means you need to ensure you have a preservative of some sort for your products.

You can colour your creams in many ways. You might like to use one of your glycerites in the mix or an infused oil. Adding oils to your cool-down phase can also change the colour. Oils like hemp seed oil will colour your cream green. This oil is heat sensitive, so needs to be added in the cool-down phase. Rose hip oil will colour your cream yellow/orange and should also be added in the cool-down phase. An infused oil of comfrey will give your cream a beautiful shade of green also. Glycerites of purple carrot, strawberry or hibiscus flowers can give your cream a beautiful pink shade. There are also essential oils like blue tansy that can give your cream a blue colour. Again, experiment here and make your own colours! This is another way of personalising your products.

Basic cream

Not everyone likes to make creams from scratch and sometimes you just don't have the time. You can add infusions, decoctions, tinctures, infused oils, glycerites and powders straight into a plain bought cream or base cream. You can only add a small amount to the cream before it is saturated and the cream starts to separate, but it can still be effective. Keep in mind if adding tinctures to creams that some people

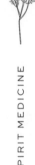
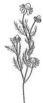

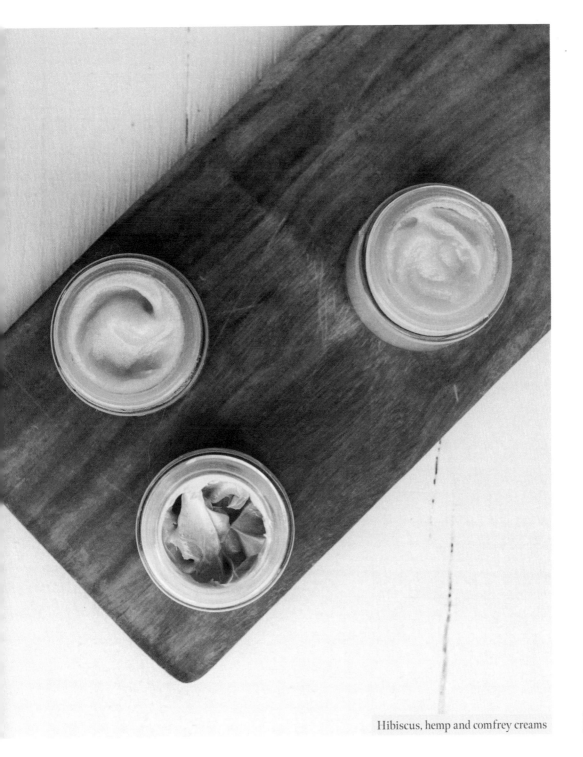

Hibiscus, hemp and comfrey creams

Comfrey oil cream

cannot tolerate the alcohol. You can heat up your tincture beforehand to evaporate the alcohol before adding. Just add it into a water bath and reduce it down to whatever you need.

The reason I like to make my creams from scratch is because a cream has a water phase and an oil phase. Once they are emulsified together, they make a cream. When you create them from scratch, you can use a herbal infusion for the water phase and an infused oil for the oil phase. This means that your cream is going to be jam packed with herbal goodness, instead of adding a few things at the end. However, since we are not making therapeutic products here, this is an entirely fine option and one I have used in the past with success.

What makes a cream different from an ointment is ointments are meant to stay on the surface of the skin longer

What makes a cream different from an ointment is ointments are meant to stay on the surface of the skin longer, so generally include more waxes, lanolin and thick oils. A cream is meant to absorb into the skin, taking with it the many water- and oil-soluble ingredients. The process of making them is basically the same; it's just the formula that is different as it now contains a water phase.

Cold-pressed creams

I love making cold-pressed creams. Why? Because they are so easy to make, and I love the textures. You also don't need a water phase, which means there is no need to use a preservative, only an antioxidant. I make a cream with just one infused oil and shea butter that turns out beautifully. Feel free to experiment with any type of plant butter and oil you like. Keep in mind: the harder the butter the thicker and harder the cream. Shea is a very soft butter, like mango butter, whereas cocoa butter is hard and really needs to be heated to melt it. Either way, if it's too hard add more oil, and if it's too soft add more butter. Experiment!

RECIPE: COLD BLENDED SHEA BUTTER CREAM

Let's start with a small batch to see how you like it. We are going to make a 20 g batch, which is a very small jar. Here are the percentages and how to work it out. Notice we are using the percentages to grams calculation, which means you are dividing by 100.

Shea butter	50%	=	50 ÷ 100 x 20 = 10 g
Infused oil	49.5%	=	49.5 ÷ 100 x 20 = 9.9 g
Vitamin E	0.5%	=	0.5 ÷ 100 x 20 = 0.1 g
	TOTAL	**=**	**20 g**

METHOD:

- *Mash up your shea butter as smooth as you can.*

- *Slowly drizzle a little of your oil into your shea butter and combine thoroughly. Keep adding a small amount until it is all incorporated into your shea butter.*

- *Add vitamin E and blend thoroughly.*

- *Jar and label.*

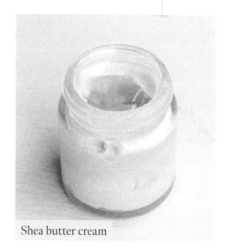

Shea butter cream

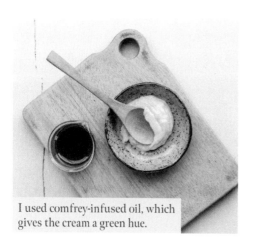

I used comfrey-infused oil, which gives the cream a green hue.

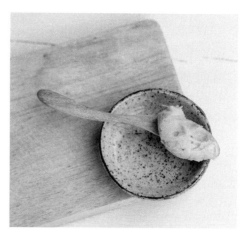

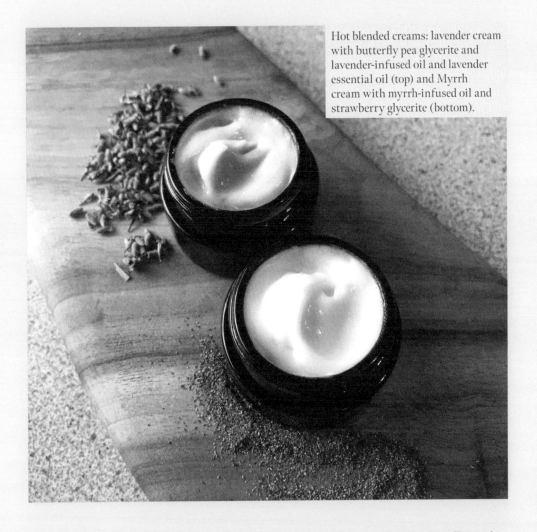

Hot blended creams: lavender cream with butterfly pea glycerite and lavender-infused oil and lavender essential oil (top) and Myrrh cream with myrrh-infused oil and strawberry glycerite (bottom).

You can see it is an easy recipe to get you started. Shea butter is normally grainy, so your cream may be slightly grainy. It doesn't affect the cream at all, but if you are concerned about it you can either keep mixing it and pushing it flat to get all the little bits out, or before you add the vitamin E (because it is heat sensitive), bring the mix up to heat in a water bath until the shea has melted and keep stirring it. Let it cool down before adding your vitamin E, and stir well again. Place it in a jar and put it in the freezer. Placing it in the freezer will make the oil and shea cool quicker, leaving less time for the shea to again crystalise. You will find though that heating it will give you a completely different consistency than non-heated. I prefer the non-heated version. Try both so you can see how they turn out.

If it ends up too liquid, add more shea. Also be aware shea is a butter, so butter and oil will be greasy but will absorb quickly. Butters are good to apply to wet skin, like when you just get out of the shower.

Hot blended creams (emulsions)

Hot blended creams, or emulsions as they are also called, take a little more work to make, but are wonderful once you get the hang of them. Essentially, there's a water phase and an oil phase, and you can use an emulsifier to bring them both together so they don't separate. We have thoroughly explored making infused oils, glycerites, infusions and decoctions, all of which can be used in both these phases, which means you can make a cream much more potent than just placing a small percentage into a finished one.

There are many types of emulsifiers on the market, so you need to find one that resonates with you and is also available where you live. The easiest to use is emulsifying wax, which is derived from coconut oil. Other emulsifiers include Olivem 1000 or 900, which are easy to use; Vegetal, also easy; lecithin (sunflower or soy, though I prefer sunflower), which can be quite tricky to work with; beeswax to a point, as it's not a strong emulsifier; or anhydrous lanolin, which has had the water removed. If you are just starting out, stick with emulsifying wax.

For this procedure, you can use two water baths or a large one big enough to fit two jugs in.

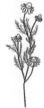

- Both the oil phase and water phase need to reach approximately the same temperature before you mix them together. The range is 65–70°C/150–160°F.

- Once they are at the right temperature, pour the water into the oil.

- Stir it continuously until the cream lowers in temperature to around 40°C/100°F, then add vitamin E, your preservative or any heat-sensitive ingredients. You can also pour it into jars at this stage, as it will still be quite liquid.

I have been making hot blended creams for decades now and have found that if you use emulsifying wax or vegetal as an emulsifier, you can heat them all up in one container instead of doing two phases. I haven't been too adventurous though with my creams. I tend to stick to a few basic formulas because they work, and what works for me might not work for your formulas. Different emulsifiers need to be worked a certain way, but give it a try anyway as it can save a lot of time. I put everything in the one jug, heat it up to close to 70°C/160°F, take it off the heat and then mix with a stick blender. I fill up my sink with cold water and place my Pyrex jug straight into it to help the mix cool down quicker. Make sure that you don't incorporate air into your cream by using the blender too fast. I just pulse it on the lowest setting and keep doing this until the cream has cooled down to 40°C/100°F to add in my last ingredients. I do find that with this method the cream is runnier at 40°C/100°F but will solidify more overnight.

Cream formulas generally equate to 30% oil and 70% water, so if you experiment, try to keep around those percentages.

RECIPE: BASIC CREAM RECIPE

Oil phase		Water phase	
Oil	24%	Water	62%
Emulsifying wax	8%	Glycerine	5%
		Citrus seed extract	1%
		TOTAL	**100%**

I have used citrus seed extract in this recipe, as it is easy to find and easy to use if you haven't made creams before. As mentioned earlier, it is an antioxidant and may also be a preservative. I have used it for many years with no issues. However, if you intend to sell commercially, you will need to use an antioxidant and a confirmed broad-spectrum preservative.

METHOD:

• *Create two water baths or a large one big enough to fit two jugs in. Place a thermometer in each jug so you can see their temperatures.*

- *Heat both the oil phase and water phase between 65–70°C/150–160°F. Just make sure they are within the range – the two don't need to be exactly the same temperature.*

- *Once they are at the right temperature slowly pour the water into the oil, which creates a beautiful reaction, and the mix then becomes opaque.*

- *Stir it continuously until the cream lowers in temperature to around 40°C/ 100°F.*

- *Pour into jars to let sit overnight. Do not put the lid on. The cream must be completely cool or mould/bacteria will grow in your product.*

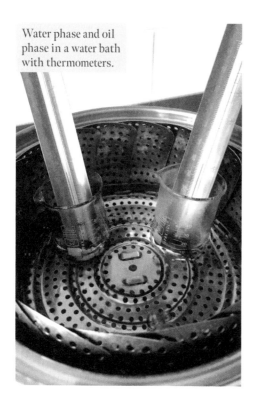

Water phase and oil phase in a water bath with thermometers.

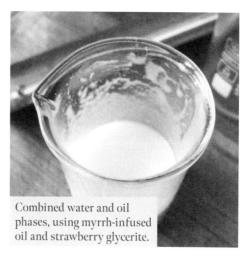

Combined water and oil phases, using myrrh-infused oil and strawberry glycerite.

This can now be used as a base cream or on its own if you have used infused oils or glycerites. Powders and essential oils can also be added to it later if you are using it as a base cream.

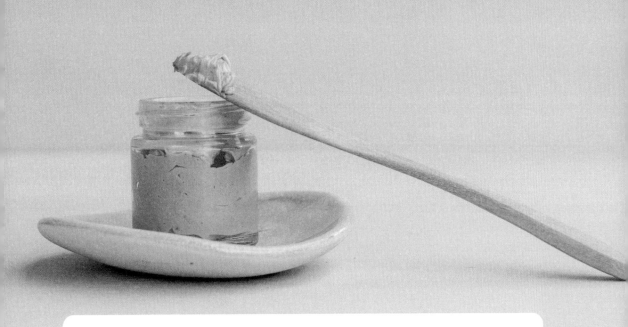

NOTE:

- *Oil can continue to get hotter after you have taken it off the stove, and it will take longer to cool, so once it is close to the minimum temperature needed take it off.*

- *Some ingredients do not handle high or prolonged temperatures, like vitamin E, rosehip oil, hemp seed oil and essential oils. These need to be added in the cool-down phase.*

- *Do not mix with a blender that incorporates air into the cream. If you use a stick blender, push it down to the bottom so it doesn't come above the surface and suck air in.*

- *The cream may look runny for quite some time, but it will start to thicken. Leave it overnight in the fridge to check how it sets properly.*

If you have created a formula that requires vitamin E, rosehip oil, hemp seed oil or essential oils, these are heat-sensitive ingredients and would be added at the 40°C /100°F mark and mixed in thoroughly. There are two ways to add these into your creams: 1) you could calculate them into your formula as percentages, or 2) use the cream you have made as a base cream to add your ingredients to at a later stage.

If you add them to your initial formula, it might look something like this. For example, I have adjusted the percentage of the oil and water to accommodate the cool-down phase percentages:

Oil phase

Oil	22%
Emulsifying wax	8%

Water phase

Water	61.5%
Glycerine	5%
Citrus seed extract	1%

Cool-down phase

Rosehip seed oil	2%
Essential oil	0.5%
TOTAL	**100%**

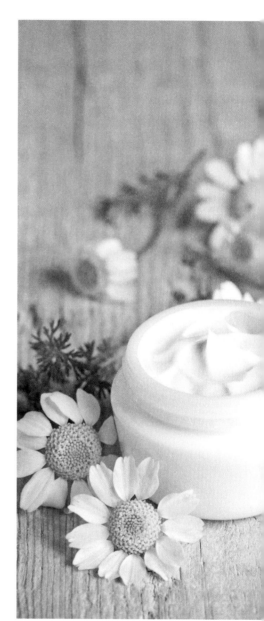

When you look at this recipe, you can see that you could potentially use an infused oil for your oil phase plus an infusion and/or glycerite in your water phase, making your cream full of botanical goodness. The oil or glycerite you decide on could be purely for colour. You can make amazing colours depending on what ingredients you use. Hemp seed oil has a beautiful fresh-looking green to it and rosehip will change your cream to a lovely yellow/ orange colour. I do find that glycerite colours can fade quicker than oil colours. There are endless possibilities for creams. If you are using pure water, use distilled water if possible.

METHOD:

- *Create two water baths or a large one big enough to fit two jugs in. Place a thermometer in each jug so you can see the temperature.*

- *Heat both the oil phase and your water phase between 65–70°C/150–160°F. Just make sure they are within the range – the two don't need to be exactly the same temperature.*

- *Once they are at the right temperature slowly pour the water into the oil, which creates a beautiful reaction, and the mix then becomes opaque.*

- *Stir it continuously until the cream lowers in temperature to around 40°C/100°F.*

- *Now add in your heat-sensitive ingredients, which are the cool-down phase ingredients.*

- *Pour into jars to let sit overnight. Do not put the lid on. The cream must be completely cool or mould/bacteria will grow in your product.*

If you want to use an antioxidant as well as a preservative your recipe might look like this:

Oil phase

Oil	24%
Emulsifying wax	8%

Water phase

Water	61%
Glycerine	5%

Cool-down phase

Vitamin E	1%
Preservative	1%
TOTAL	**100%**

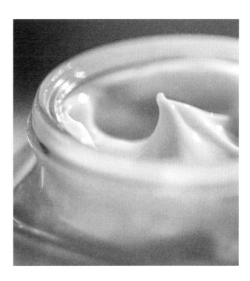

Follow the method above to make the cream with this one extra step: to add your preservative, make sure everything is in the cream that needs to be in there. Take a small amount of your product out to test its pH. Check with your preservative supplier what the suggested range of the pH needs to be for your specific preservative. Plantaserv M, which I use, has to have a pH between 3 and 8. The skin generally needs to have products that range between 5 and 5.5. If you add a preservative to a cream where the pH is too high or too low for it, it can make the preservative unstable. Preservatives can also lower the pH of your cream – this is why you also need to check the pH of your cream after the preservative has been added. Sounds a bit tricky, but once you get the hang of it you'll be fine.

Measuring pH

If you plan to make creams for commercial sale, it is important you measure the pH of your products. You cannot measure the pH of balms and ointments because they have no water content.

When starting out all you need are some paper pH strips. These are easily obtainable over the internet and don't cost much at all. Try to avoid the yellow litmus paper ones as they are not very accurate. They are more for soap. If you want to advance in this area you can buy a pH meter. I have heard they can be a bit tricky to use, but if you want to become a professional at creams I suggest you invest in one.

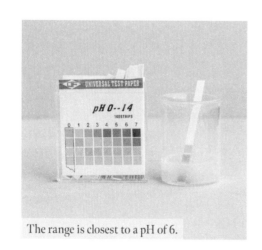

The range is closest to a pH of 6.

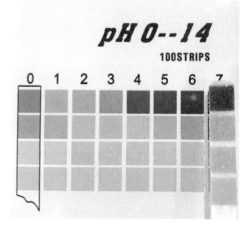

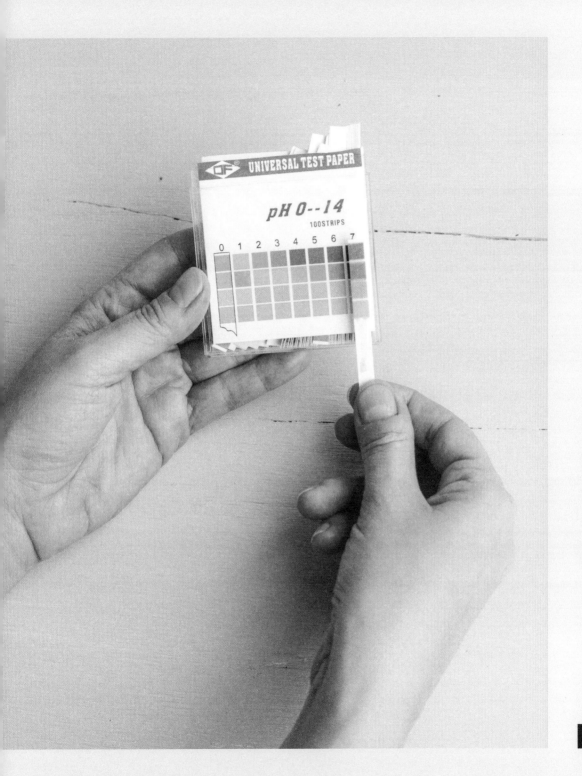

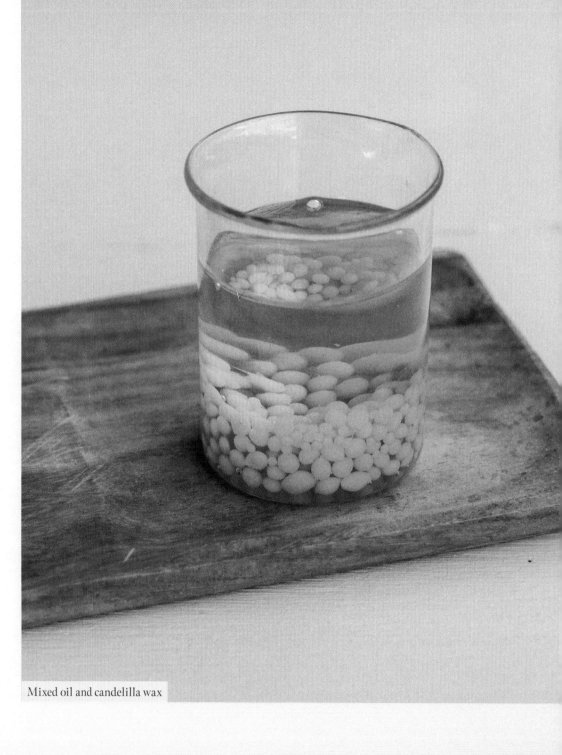

Mixed oil and candelilla wax

Testing your sample

First place 1 g of your sample into a glass beaker and add about 9 g of distilled water. Stir the sample well and dip your paper into the mix. Then check the pH on the packaging.

If you are going to add a preservative to your product, check that the pH is within the range needed for the preservative to work effectively. If it is, you can add your preservative to the product. If it isn't, you will need to adjust it. When you add your preservative it can change the pH of your product, so it is a good practice to check the product's pH again using a 1 g sample. If the cream is within the 5–5.5 range, then you are fine. If it is higher or lower, you can do the following to bring it into the right measurement. You will also need to do this before adding your preservative to your cream if the pH isn't within the range needed for your preservative.

Adjusting the pH

There are a few solutions you can use to adjust pH. I like to keep it simple and just use two: one for raising the pH – sodium bicarbonate – and one for lowering it – citric acid.

- Use 10% either sodium bicarbonate or citric acid with 90% distilled water.
- This would look like 1 g + 9 g.

Only a few drops are needed. You might like to keep these in glass dropper bottles, but they can only be kept for around a week.

So, essentially, add either a drop of your sodium bicarbonate or citric acid mix to your product to either raise or lower the pH. Keep testing the pH until you have it within the range needed.

> **NOTE:** *changing the pH of your product can make the colour change. Sometimes aloe vera can go pink, butterfly pea changes from blue to purple to pink. This can work as an advantage and sometimes not.*

Here is a recipe for lavender cream that I make from my own infused lavender oil and butterfly pea glycerite. The butterfly pea glycerite is a magnificent blue, but when we combine the mix it becomes a diluted blue – then when the preservative is added it changes to a lavender colour, which is perfect for this cream! Although being a glycerite, this colour doesn't last long.

RECIPE: LAVENDER CREAM

Oil phase

Lavender-infused oil	23.5%
Emulsifying wax	8%

Water phase

Water	60.5%
Butterfly pea glycerite	5%

Cool-down phase

Vitamin E	1%
Lavender essential oil	1%
Preservative	1%
TOTAL	**100%**

METHOD: as per previous method on page 149.

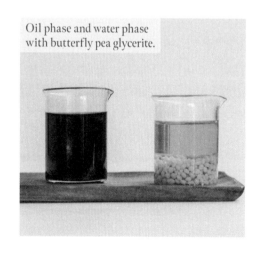

Oil phase and water phase with butterfly pea glycerite.

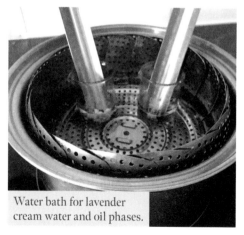

Water bath for lavender cream water and oil phases.

Sprays

Facial or room sprays are another favourite of mine. Not only are they easy to make, they can make you or your room feel and smell amazing.

Some keep in the fridge well, or you might like to add a preservative or alcohol. If you are making a room spray, keep in mind the fine particles of the spray can be inhaled, so be aware of anything you put in there and potential toxicities.

Floral waters or hydrosols are great to use here and can be purchased readily. If you make your own, kudos to you. Ones that you purchase generally have preservatives already added to them, but you can buy some that are 100% pure. Essential oils work great in sprays. Again, if you make your own hydrosols and your own essential oils, these sprays would be amazing to make as you would be so close to your plant spirit through the whole process. You might want to look at purchasing a copper alembic still for this.

Room sprays are 100% liquid. They are generally one part water, one part witch hazel/vodka and anywhere from 10 to 40 drops of essential oil, sometimes more. I am no authority on the use of essential oils, so I like to play it safe.

As oil and water don't mix, the essential oils will sit on the surface of the water without the use of a solubiliser or ethanol. A solubiliser helps dissolve the oils into the water. There are a few solubilisers you can use, including:

- **Alcohol** – this needs to be at least 75% ethanol (grain alcohol) and up to 95%. Unfortunately, vodka doesn't really cut it as it is normally 60% water, which means 40% alcohol.

- **Polysorbate** – Symbio®solv XC is a good natural choice here.

Some DIY sites will say you can use vodka or witch hazel, however, these are not really strong enough to disperse the oils through the water or preserve the mix properly. Witch hazel normally has a percentage of around 14% alcohol already in it, but this is still not enough.

If you use ethanol, you have the added benefit of not needing a preservative. I suggest, again, that if you are going to sell your products commercially, invest in a recognised preservative. You also need to ensure your preservative is water soluble.

The preservatives already mentioned earlier in the book are all water soluble so are good choices here, and again you only need 1%.

Sprays using essential oils also need to be in dark glass bottles because essential oils can destroy plastic and light can degrade the oils.

There are many ways to make a room spray depending on what ingredients you use. If you don't use polysorbate solubiliser, you can use the following recipe.

RECIPE: SPRAY WITHOUT SOLUBILISER

Water	72%
Ethanol	25%
Essential oils	3%
TOTAL	**100%**

METHOD:

- *Place your ethanol straight into your glass bottle and add your essential oils to it. Mix it all around and leave to stand for around 45 minutes to an hour.*

- *Slowly add your water phase. This could be a hydrosol, distilled water or witch hazel.*

- *Shake well and label.*

Alternatively, you can use a solubiliser. You use one part essential oils to one part solubiliser. Always add your essential oils to the solubiliser first, then add your water, alcohol/witch hazel and/or preservative.

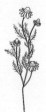

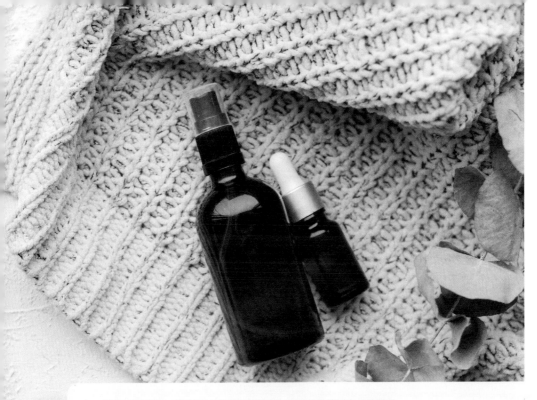

RECITE: SPRAY WITH SOLUBILISER

Liquid	93% *(this can be made up of distilled water, hydrosol, witch hazel, alcohol or an infusion)*
Essential oils	3% *(you can go up to 5%, but also adjust your solubiliser to 5% and minus 4% from your liquid portion so everything still adds up to 100%)*
Solubiliser	3%
Preservative	1%
TOTAL	**100%**

METHOD:

- *Place the essential oils and solubiliser either straight into your bottle or into a glass beaker/jug to mix. It is important to mix these together first before adding your liquid.*

- *Add the liquid phase and check your pH.*

- *If the pH is within the right range for your chosen preservative, add your preservative and then mix well to combine it all and label.*

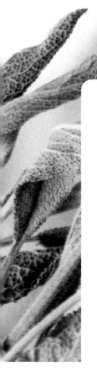

RECIPE: WHITE SAGE SPRAY

If you grow your own white sage, this is a lovely spray to use around the home to help cleanse the air and work with the sacred white sage plant spirit. I don't use white sage essential oil at this time due to the controversy surrounding the over-use of this sacred plant. If we grow it ourselves we are honouring it, and it will also be sustainable for our products. In the infusion of white sage there will be a lot of plant matter, so it will be hard to preserve for a length of time. I will therefore add ethanol as well as a preservative. Also, because I am not using essential oils, I do not need a solubiliser.

White sage infusion	74%
Ethanol	25%
Preservative	1%
TOTAL	**100%**

METHOD:

• *Make an infusion of dried white sage in distilled water.*

• *Add ethanol and preservative. Add to a glass spray bottle, shake well and label.*

• *If you can't obtain ethanol, do try as high a percentage vodka as possible. You might like to increase the alcohol percentage and decrease the infusion amount. As long as you have the preservative and some alcohol, it will preserve. It is hard to determine how long it will last, so it is always good to keep checking your spray for any nasties.*

Facial sprays

Another great way to use sprays is for the face. They make you feel refreshed, the smell is uplifting and some can have a toning effect on the skin.

You can use aloe vera juice on its own as well as witch hazel and rose hydrosol. Apple cider vinegar is also great for the skin, so you can use your vinegar infusions here (generally at 5% of your liquid phase). Keep in mind that alcohol is drying to the skin, so research your essential oils to ensure they are safe for use on the skin.

Dried herbs

Teas

As already discussed, infusions or teas are the most basic form of working with dried herbs. There are so many variations and creating your own is rewarding. The connection you make to a plant by growing it yourself, harvesting it, drying it and then drinking it is one you will appreciate. Even pulling dandelions from your lawn and drying them out to use the roots as a tea is so rewarding! Ensure you know what plant you are picking. Dandelions are so versatile; you can use the whole plant. The root is known for helping the liver, while the leaves are a diuretic, which benefits the kidneys. This simple little garden weed has tremendous value – a lesson in itself, representing joy, happiness and letting go.

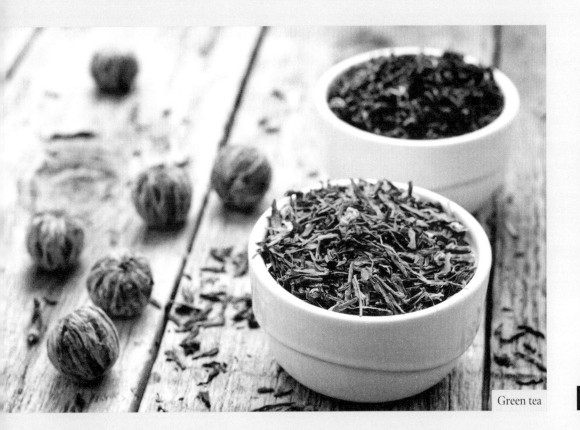

Green tea

You can also create beautiful steam inhalations with your herbs just like your infusions, but you inhale the aroma instead of drinking it. This works great with fragrant herbs. Remember to check that your plant is safe to do this with.

Bath teas

Bath teas are another lovely way of working with herbs/plants. Flowers make great bath teas because they look beautiful floating on the top of the water: dried or fresh rose petals, even dandelion flowers! Generally, with bath teas you would place your herbs into a large muslin bag and tie it to the tap so the water can run through it, but you can also place the plant matter into your bath if you desire. Oats are great to add to the bath to soothe irritated skin (place in a bag), and you could use a mix of plants for various reasons. You could also make up a strong infusion and pour it into your bath water, like chamomile for example.

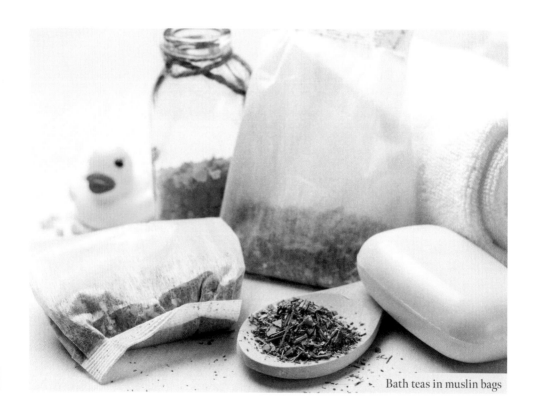

Bath teas in muslin bags

I make a strong infusion of rosemary, let it cool and pour it through my hair after I have conditioned it to make it nice and shiny. The smell as you pour it over your head is beautiful. This is one versatile herb you should definitely consider growing yourself – it makes a fabulous addition to your bath as well. Its spirit medicine is about cleansing, peace and purification. It also makes great smudge sticks!

Foot baths are also a great idea with herbs, especially for those with cold feet – or if your feet are swollen from the heat, you can place them in cold water. It is well known that the body absorbs herbal applications through the feet that benefit the entire body, so again be mindful as to what you put your feet into. Peppermint or cedarwood are great to use for tired feet or poor circulation. Mint's spirit medicine is also about clarity, focus and calm, while cedarwood is helpful for balancing and grounding and is great for meditation.

Eye baths and gargles are another way you can use your herbal infusion. Again, check that your plant is suitable. Chamomile and calendula make great eye baths, and sage is well known as a throat gargle.

Sachets

Herbal pillows or sachets have been used for centuries. These small, simple fabric bags or pillows can be placed under or in your bed pillow so you inhale the smell of the herbs

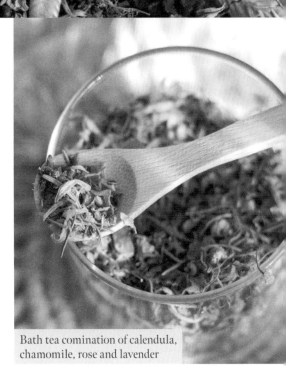

Bath tea comination of calendula, chamomile, rose and lavender

Chamomile and calendula make great eye baths, and sage is well known as a throat gargle

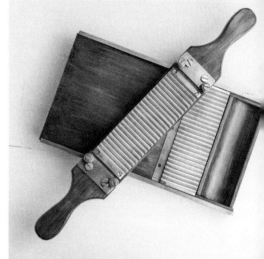

throughout the night. You can also carry them on you. They range from simple lavender herbal pillows to help with sleep to Chinese sachets with herbal formulas to help with a range of conditions. They are easy to make and are a great way to work with dried, scented herbs. Mugwort, for instance, is known for its visionary or dreaming medicine, so putting mugwort in a fabric sachet to place in your pillow is a great form of Plant Spirit Medicine. Call on the plant spirit to help you dream of an answer or for inspiration. Drinking the tea is also an option.

Powders, pills and capsules

I love making pills from powdered herbs. They are super simple and allow you to have them on hand when needed. Honey is generally used as the binder and also helps preserve them. It's as simple as grinding your herbs to a powder and adding a little honey until the consistency can be rolled into a ball. You can also coat them in cocoa or slippery elm powder to stop them from sticking together. I find I don't need to if I don't use too much honey.

First grind your herb/plant down to a powder. Coffee grinders are great for this, especially when doing small batches, or you can use a small blender. I've tried using a mortar and pestle, but the little stringy bits don't break down enough.

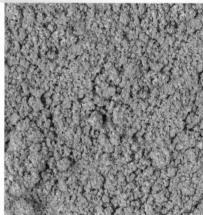

Call on the plant spirit to help you dream of an answer or for inspiration

I also have an antique pill roller. These were used in the 1800s in apothecaries and pharmacies to make their pills up. They are so much fun to use!

Roll your mix into a ball and place the paddle with the wood side down onto the ball and roll it out to a long thin strip. If you don't have a pill roller, roll the ball out to a long thin strip, then chop pieces off and roll into balls.

Once it is rolled evenly, turn the paddle over so the brass plates align, place your rolled herb mix up to the plates, slide the plates over the mix a few times then let the balls roll out into the catcher. I have used a Chinese herbal formula for these pills, Xiao Yao San (for stress), and you could also make Bao He Wan (for digestive issues). These are great if you don't like the taste of herb decoctions.

You can create your own with single herbs or a mix, and this is again another way of digesting your herb/plant. Always check first whether your plant is edible – if you are unsure, then don't ingest it. At the end of the day, it's not essential to include a plant in your diet – you can access the Plant Spirit Medicine without it. If it is safe to ingest, then also ensure you research the recommended dosage and/or potential side effects.

Another recipe I like to make is slippery elm balls.

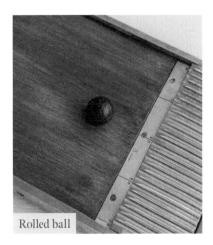
Rolled ball

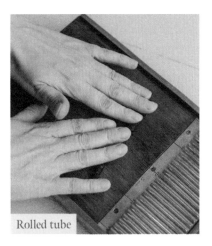
Rolled tube

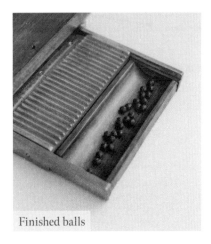
Finished balls

RECIPE: SLIPPERY ELM BALLS

Slippery elm bark powder is an amazing herb to help with digestive issues. It is a nutritive to the digestive tract and it also helps coat it, which makes it great for irritated digestive systems. It is a bulking fibre as well, so good for constipation and diarrhoea. Plus there's the added benefit of being able to work with the slippery elm tree as a spirit medicine, which is known as a great protector. Here's how to make the pills.

METHOD:

- *Place a tablespoon of slippery elm in a bowl or mortar and pestle.*

- *Add around a teaspoon of honey and combine well, adding more honey if needed.*

- *The mix needs to reach a consistency that isn't overly sticky, but sticky enough to form into little balls. Roll each one and, if needed, you can roll them in a little extra slippery elm or some cocoa to keep them from sticking to one another. Keep washing your hands to stop the balls from sticking to them.*

- *Let the balls dry out, and place them in an airtight container for whenever you need them. Depending on how big you make them, normally the dose is about a small teaspoon of slippery elm in a glass of water two to three times a day, so use roughly a teaspoon of the balls. Make them small enough to swallow whole!*

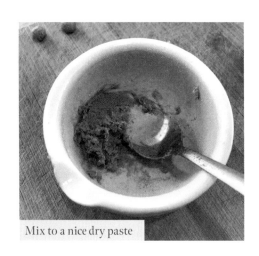

Mix to a nice dry paste

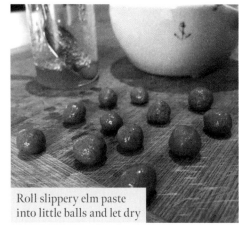

Roll slippery elm paste into little balls and let dry

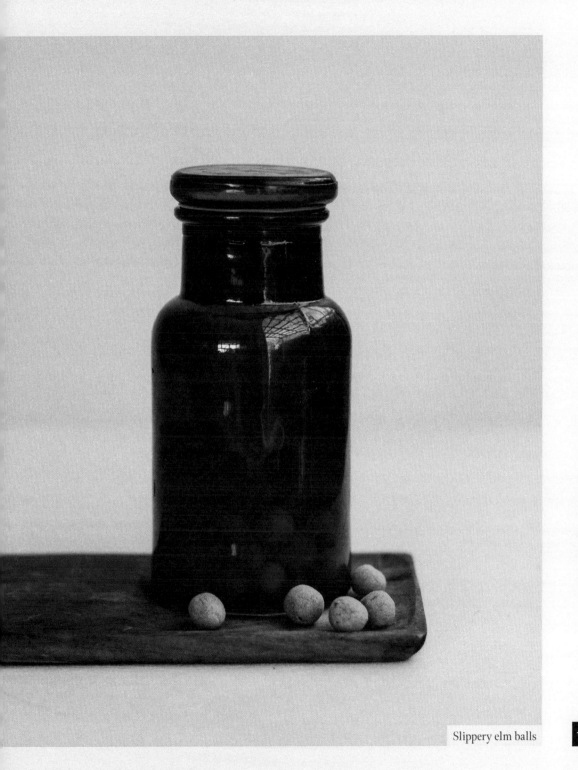

Slippery elm balls

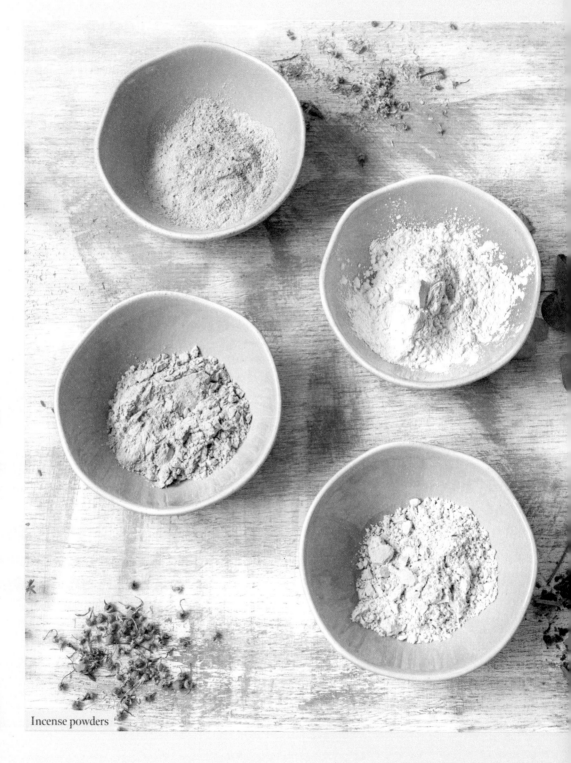

Incense powders

Incense

Incense has played an incredibly important role through the years as a medicine, whether spiritual, emotional or physical. Chinese herbal remedies have been made into medicinal incense to help with physical conditions when burned, resins are used in ritual all around the world, and we are all familiar with incense sticks for home use.

I am certainly no expert on incense making, so I will leave that to others who are as that could be a whole book by itself, but there are a few methods you might like to consider to get you started. It is a really rewarding process.

Loose incense: powdered herbs and resins can be placed on non-toxic charcoal bases or incense warmers to help release their beautiful aromas. Creating a loose blend is an easy process.

- Always ensure you weigh everything so you can replicate it if it works out well.

- Grind your herbs or plant matter down to small granules or a powder. Grinding resins, as previously discussed, can be difficult. Freeze the resin before trying to grind it or buy it already ground.

- Mix small amounts of your powders together and heat to smell if the aroma smells good. Don't waste large amounts. Once you have found a good mix, bottle it and label.

- Store it in a dark, cool place. The incense will mature the longer you leave it as all the plants merge together or 'synergise' – 48 hours is a good start.

NOTE: *this is not a combustible incense, meaning it won't burn on its own unless you use only a very thin layer, hence why we need to burn it on a non-toxic charcoal disk or in an incense warmer.*

If we want a loose incense that can burn by itself like the ones used in incense trails or for making incense cones, we first need to add makko powder, and the powder must be fine sieved. The higher the quality makko you use the better the smell and function of your incense.

Incense trails were used in China and Japan as a form of time keeping, as well as for their beauty and in ritual. Essentially, powdered incense is placed in patterns or trails on top of white chaff ash within a bowl. The incense is then lit, and it burns from one end of the trail to the other. They are incredibly beautiful and require you to be still and have patience in making them. This is a great addition to any ritual or honouring of the plant/s you choose to create your incense from.

Adding makko to your loose incense is again a bit of trial and error, because it all depends on what you have in your loose incense. If it is mainly wood or herbs, the percentage of makko needed will range from 5–30%, but if you use a high proportion of resins you will need anything from 40–90%. Again, we can use a calculation for working out how much we need.

Weight of your loose incense x percentage of makko needed = amount of makko you need to add to your loose incense.

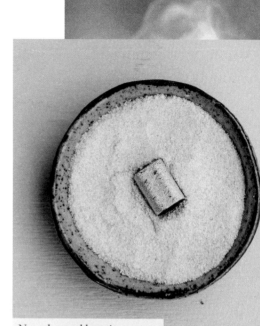
Non-charcoal burning square

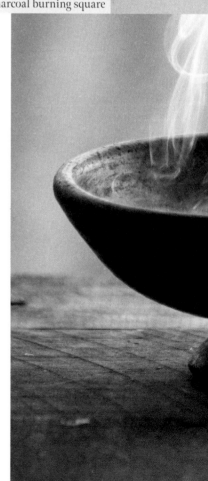

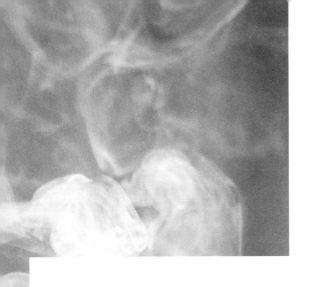

If it goes out you will know you need more makko; if it burns too fast you will need less

e.g. 40 g of incense x 30% makko − (40 x 0.3) = 12 g of makko required to add to your loose incense mix.

Combine both together and do a test to make sure it burns by making a small trail of incense in some ash and lighting it. It needs to burn slow and steady. If it goes out you will know you need more makko; if it burns too fast you will need less. Make sure you record how much you add or need to subtract, so that when you reach the right balance you can replicate it again. Once you have reached the right balance of incense to makko you can use it as is or you can make it into cones.

Now that you also know the measurements of each you can create a formula in percentages, which means going back to our calculations:

e.g.

Loose incense	40 g	
Makko	12 g	
TOTAL	**52 g**	

Convert weight to percentages formula:
(weight x 100 ÷ total weight of original formula)

Loose incense	40 g x 100 ÷ 52	=	77%
Makko	12 g x 100 ÷ 52	=	23%
TOTAL	**52 g**	**=**	**100%**

Now you can replicate your incense mix to any quantities.

Making incense cones

Take a portion of your loose incense and makko mix.

Place in a bowl and very slowly add warm distilled water or hydrosol (if using a hydrosol, ensure it is 100% with no preservatives added). We are aiming for a dough mix, so knead the water in slowly and don't let it get too wet. The dough needs to be able to stick together when squeezed but not have water dripping out of it and no cracks when it holds together.

Once kneaded well, leave the dough in the bowl overnight but cover it with a damp cloth.

The next day all you need to do is take small amounts and shape them into a cone or your desired shape – taking into consideration the thicker you make it, the harder it may be to burn. You can also roll the dough out flat and cut into shapes using small cutters, which would then resemble more of a traditional incense tablet. Traditionally, they would normally be heated next to a charcoal disc or on an incense warmer, but if you make them big enough they can be lit like an incense cone to burn by themselves.

Dry your shapes on a tray with wax paper. If you can put this inside a large paper bag do so, but if not find some paper to cover them. You want them to dry out without losing their smell, but not be too enclosed that they go mouldy before drying.

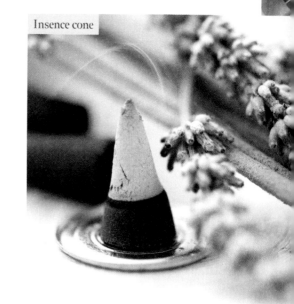

Insence cone

Once fully dry, keep them in an airtight dark container and label.

If they don't end up working out, you can crush them up, fix the mix by adding more makko or loose incense and repeat the process.

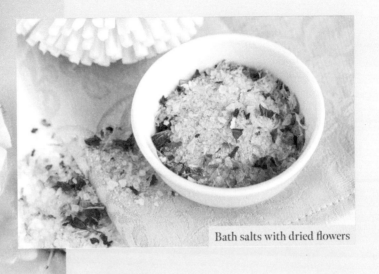

Bath salts with dried flowers

Baths

Baths are becoming a bit of a rare commodity these days. Showers have easily taken over because everything is about rushing and getting things done quickly. In some places, there is a need to conserve water too, so running a luxurious bath every night isn't on the cards for everyone. But when was the last time you took time out of your routine and treated yourself to a bath, when you slowed down and really relaxed? Sometimes it's hard to just relax because we have been pushing ourselves for so long. Having a bath using Plant Spirit Medicine then is the perfect chance to slow down enough to form a relationship with the plant spirits. If a bath isn't an option for you, consider a small foot bath. You can even use a bowl or a bucket. Foot baths are great for those winter days when you have cold feet or if you have achy, painful feet or ankles.

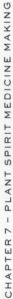

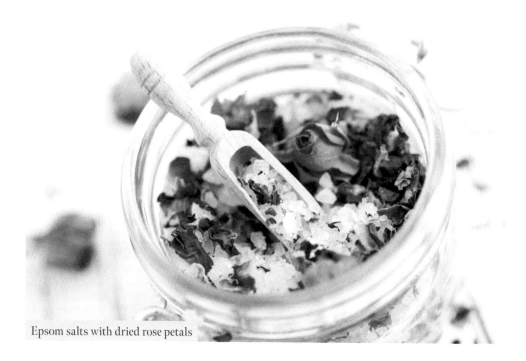
Epsom salts with dried rose petals

We have already discussed bath teas, so we have to decide on what we want from our bath and plant interaction. Do we just need to relax and slow down? Maybe choose a nice relaxing herb like lavender or hops. Maybe we want to pamper ourselves and give ourselves some love. Rose petals or vervain might be beneficial here.

Bath salts

We've all seen gorgeous jars full of mixtures of herbs and bath salts – a beautiful addition to any bath but also an opportunity to relax the body and work with the plant spirits.

Epsom salts are a well-known salt for relaxing tired, aching muscles, but we can also use rock or sea salt. Do not use normal table salt. You can also use milk powder as this is soothing for your skin and essential oils can be mixed in to give it a divine smell. I like to save and dry my own rose petals exactly for these type of creations (as long as they are spray free).

Bath salts are the easiest thing to make. It's as simple as placing all your dried ingredients in a bowl and mixing them all together. Place them in a nice glass jar and sprinkle them in the water when you need them.

RECIPE: BASIC BATH SALTS

Epsom salts	40%
Pink salt or sea salt	25% (pink salt gives it a nice mixed colour)
Bicarb soda	23%
Essential oils	2%
Dried rose petals	10% (or any flower/herb of your choice)
TOTAL	**100%**

METHOD:

- *Place the Epsom salts, pink salt or sea salt and bicarb in a mixing bowl and then add the essential oils. Combine thoroughly.*

- *Add the dried rose petals, mix again and pour into a glass jar.*

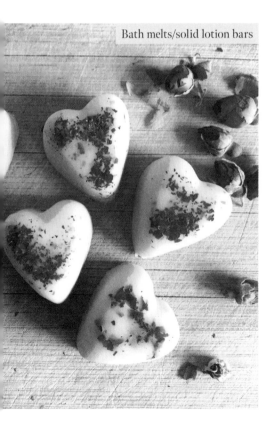

Bath melts/solid lotion bars

Bath melts or solid lotion bars

These are literally my favourite products to make. If you love chocolate as much as me, you will love making them too. These bars are based on cocoa butter and they smell of chocolate. That's not the only reason I love making them, though. I participated in a cacao ceremony many years ago and it was simply amazing. I met the cacao plant spirit, and it is something I will never forget. After the ceremony I left quickly so I could go and draw the being I had just encountered. The spirit had no mouth or nose but communicated telepathically with me. I felt it to be a female energy, but it encompassed both male and female. To this day I'm not sure what it told me, but it showed me around an incredibly old and sacred forest of the most ancient and tallest trees I've ever seen. The scale was absolutely enormous and doesn't exist in this physical reality. I felt such a sacred connection to this spirit that I always enjoy working with and respecting the beauty of the cacao tree and plant spirit now.

What are solid lotion bars and bath melts? They are the same thing – a beautiful blend of natural butters for the skin, with infused oils or essential oils and dried herbs incorporated into them. You can simply drop one in your bath, let it melt, smell the beautiful aromas and feel the nourishment of the butters on your skin, while the dried herbs dance around the surface of the water; or rub one along your skin after a shower, let it melt, then rub it in. They can make your bath a little oily, which equates to slippery, so bear that in mind! They can also be tied up in a little muslin bag to hang from the bath tap or to float in the bath.

Here's a basic recipe that is really easy to make. For the oil component, you can use any infused oil. These bath melts do melt in hot temperatures, so I generally make them heading into winter or I store them in the fridge. The cocoa butter is what gives them their hardness, so if they are too hard reduce the amount of cocoa butter, or if they are too soft add more.

RECIPE: BASIC BATH MELT

Cocoa butter	70%
Mango butter	20% *(you can use shea butter or another soft butter here)*
Infused oil	8%
Vitamin E	1%
Essential oils	1%
TOTAL	**100%**

EXTRAS NEEDED:

- **Dried herbs/flowers** (optional)

- **Silicon mould** – *these can be silicon ice cube trays or silicone chocolate moulds. Do not use normal plastic moulds as the heat from the mixture can shrink and melt the mould.*

First you need to work out how much your mould will take. Pour some oil into one of the sections in the mould right to the top and then pour it into a beaker to weigh. *(Make sure you weigh the beaker on the scales first, so you aren't adding the weight of your beaker to the oil.)* This weight measurement now tells you how much in weight you need to fill one mould. You then multiply it by how many bars you want to make.

For instance, my heart mould has 14 hearts in the one mould. Each heart will take 14 g of oil. So if I only need to make three hearts I multiply 14 x 3, which equals 42 g. I now have the total amount needed to make three heart bars.

With the percentages above, your recipe now would take the following:

Cocoa butter	29.4 g
Mango butter	8.4 g
Infused oil	3.36 g
Vitamin E	0.42 g
Essential oils	0.42 g
TOTAL	**42 g**

METHOD:

- *You can get your mould ready first by placing some dried herbs in the bottom of each mould. This ensures they are on the top of your bar when you push it out later. For this recipe I have used lavender flowers, with lavender-infused oil and lavender essential oil.*

- *Place the cocoa and mango butters plus your infused oil into a Pyrex jug in a water bath and heat until melted.*

- *When the mix has cooled to around 50°C/120°F, add your vitamin E and essential oils and pour into your moulds. Take care when pouring to keep your herbs in place if you want them just on the top of your bath melt, or you can pour a little in first to stop them from floating around and then fill them.*

- *Place them in the fridge or freezer to harden then store them in the fridge or wrap them in some greaseproof paper.*

If you live in a warm climate, you can add some wax to your lotion bars to help them stay solid. I add candelilla wax to mine at a percentage of 20%, but you can play with that percentage. Here is how I would adjust the recipe.

RECIPE: LAVENDER SOLID LOTION BAR WITH WAX

Cocoa butter	50%
Mango butter	20%
Candelilla wax	20%
Lavender-infused oil	8%
Vitamin E	1%
Lavender essential oil	1%
TOTAL	**100%**

METHOD: as per previous steps. Add your candelilla wax to the butters and oil and melt them all together.

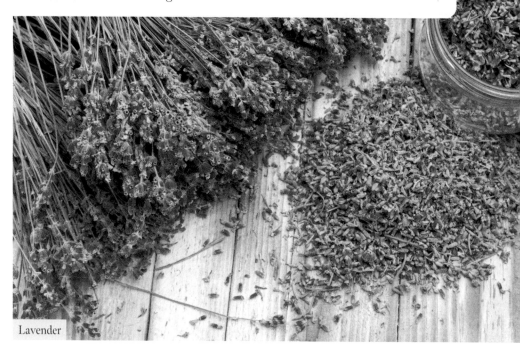

Lavender

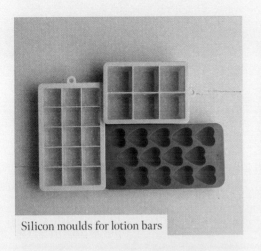

Silicon moulds for lotion bars

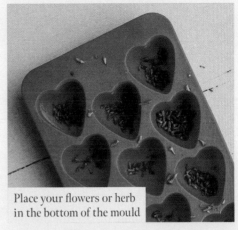

Place your flowers or herb in the bottom of the mould

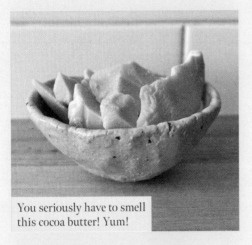

You seriously have to smell this cocoa butter! Yum!

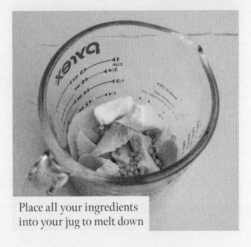

Place all your ingredients into your jug to melt down

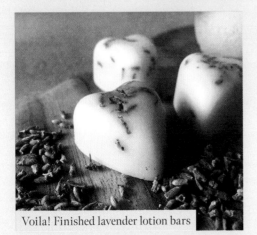

Voila! Finished lavender lotion bars

I add candelilla wax to mine at a percentage of 20%, but you can play with that percentage

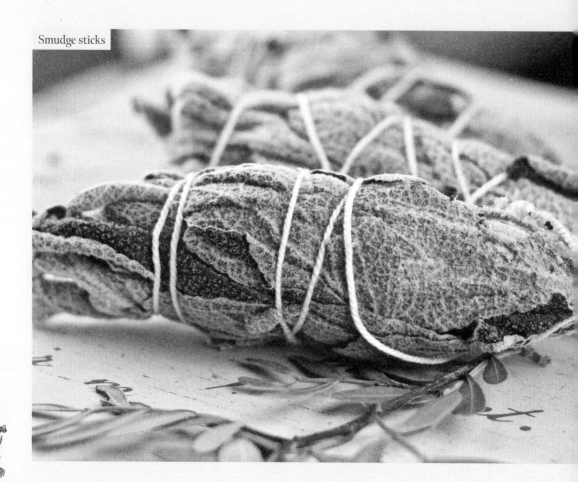

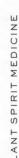

Smudge sticks

Smudge sticks are known for being made from white sage. Smudge is used to clear the air of unwanted energies, so to speak, but has also been found to have antibacterial qualities. As has already been discussed, white sage is now being grossly over-harvested due to its popularity, and indigenous peoples are asking for its use to be reduced as it is sacred to their societies.

We must look at the sustainability of any plant we use. Population numbers on earth are growing exponentially and nothing is really sustainable if we don't all play our individual part. For this reason I grow my own white sage, thus making my products sustainable. I not only create a relationship with the white sage plant spirit, I also respect it by finding a sustainable source.

Besides, there are many other plants that can be used as smudge. There are many native plants in your area that could be used. We need to always push our thinking further and ask ourselves and spirit if there is something else that can be used in its place.

Other herbs you might like to use as smudge are common sage, mugwort, rosemary, lavender, cedar, thyme, yarrow or sweetgrass. There's no doubt many more, so investigate what is local to your area.

METHOD:

You can bind your herbs the day you harvest them or when they are dry. Tie them tightly when they are fresh because they shrink in size once the water content has evaporated, which makes the string holding them together loose. If you tie them together when they are dry it can be hard to tie them tightly together because they are so stiff. Experiment with what works for you. If you do tie up fresh herbs, make sure they get lots of airflow so they dry well in the middle instead of growing mould. Tie them up and hang them in a window or outside.

- *Cut your stems/branches as long as you need, aiming for as many leaves as possible.*

- *Cut off a good metre or so of a natural-fibre string/cotton and find the middle of the string. Place the middle of the string onto the bottom of the stems/branches and tie them firmly at the bottom.*

- *You should now have two pieces of string to tie the bundle from the bottom. Wrap one string going one way up the bundle and the other piece of string up it in the opposite direction so they end up overlapping as they travel up the bundle. Once they reach the top, tie them in a knot and trim the string.*

Once dry, your smudge stick is ready to use. All you need to do is light the end and guide the smoke around the room, normally with the use of a large feather or smudge fan. Be careful of the burning embers as you blow the smoke around. Place it in a large shell or dish with ash in it once you are done smudging.

All you need to do is light the end and guide the smoke around the room . . .

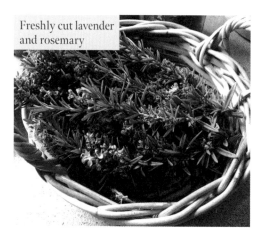

Freshly cut lavender and rosemary

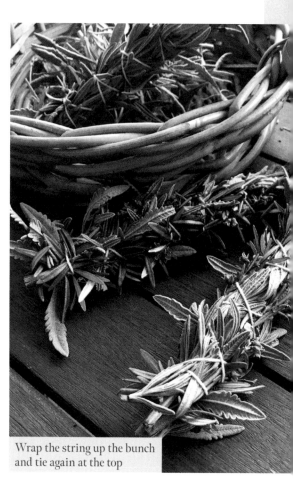

Wrap the string up the bunch and tie again at the top

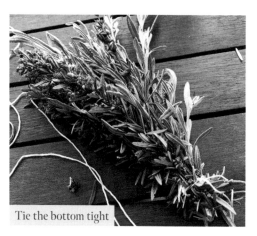

Tie the bottom tight

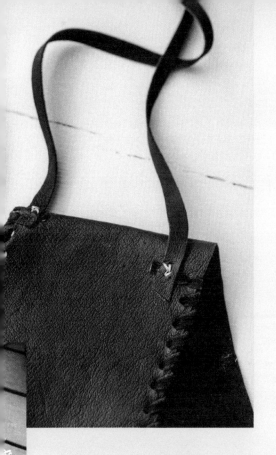

Medicine bag making

Plant Spirit Medicine making doesn't always have to be about physical products to use; it can be as simple as creating a medicine bag for yourself or someone else. I seriously could have a hundred of these bags, I love them so much! You can make them yourself from material or leather, and there really are no limits. Make them as simple or elaborate as you like. You can also honour animal spirits by adorning them with feathers, bones or furs as you see fit. I like to use found objects like feathers or naturally shed snake skins but have on occasion repurposed fur that was once used

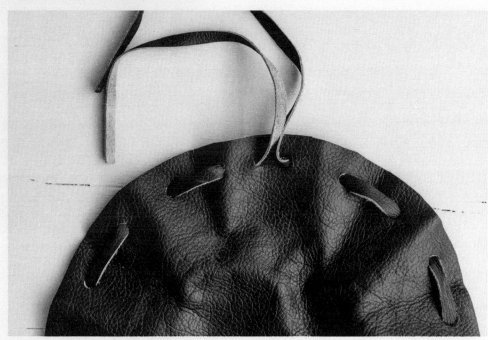

as a fur jacket. By working in ritual you can call the animal spirit back to the fur and ask for its permission. You show the spirit what you wish to create with it and how you will actually honour its spirit for a beautiful purpose. I know this is a touchy subject for some, so just do what feels right for you. When you ask permission and work with respect and honour you will know if it is right.

What can you put in a medicine bag? Anything you want! If you are working with a specific plant spirit you might like to place a part of it in your medicine bag to carry with you at all times. You can place resins, leaves, barks and flowers in them. You can combine them and even add crystals. Each medicine bag can have its own purpose, and once you feel it has done its job you simply change what's in there.

Here are a few simple medicine bag templates you can use to make your own medicine bag.

Leather bag

When working with leather, the good thing is you don't have to edge it in any way to stop it from fraying. This makes leather medicine bags quick to make and patterns are a lot easier. You can even cut from one strip of leather. Soft leather is best. Find a place that sells offcuts or go to your local second-hand shop and see if they have a cheap leather jacket. I always like to recycle and repurpose where possible.

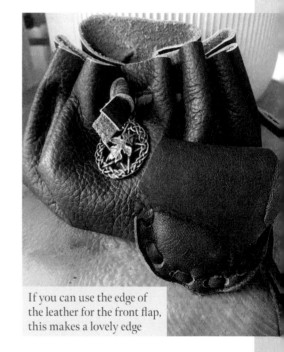

If you can use the edge of the leather for the front flap, this makes a lovely edge

There are a couple of quick ways to make a leather medicine bag. Pictured at right are two bags of my own that I made myself. The green bag (**style 1**) is for around my neck and the larger one (**style 2**) is for on a belt. Both can be made without the use of a sewing machine – all you need is some scissors and a hole punch.

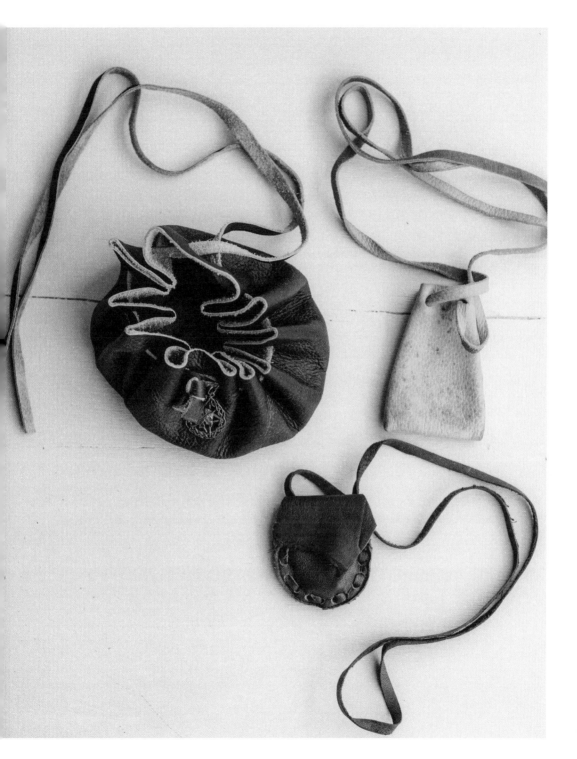

METHOD 1:

- *Cut two pieces of leather – one for the back and one for the front.*

- *While they are together, punch holes around the curved part only, not the front flap. Do them together so the holes match up.*

- *Cut a long strip of leather that is the same width or slightly bigger than the holes you just punched out.*

- *Thread them through the holes. You can do this two ways.*

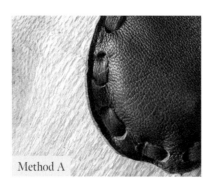
Method A

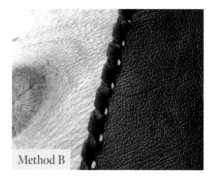
Method B

- *Cut the ties so that you can sew them onto the back of the bag out of the way. Now cut another long strip of leather to attach to the back of the bag for its strap. Make it as long as you need it, so decide if it will be a necklace or if you need it for any other purpose. Sew this onto the back over the top of the ties that you sewed in place.*

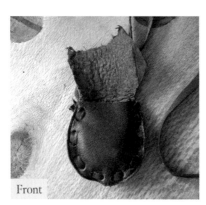
Front

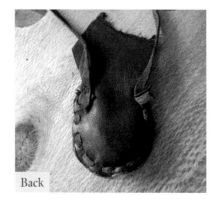
Back

FOLD LINE

- - - - - - - -

BACK   FRONT

The second style of leather bag is simple to make, and you can customise the inside as well with a wood-burning pyrograph tool.

METHOD 2:

- *Starting with a circle of leather, punch holes around the outside and thread a small thin strip of leather through the circles. When you pull them together the bag pulls closed.*

- *It's important that you punch an even number of holes around the circle so that when you thread it up both ends come out at the same place.*

- *You can also thread the leather ties through a bead to keep the bag closed if needed.*

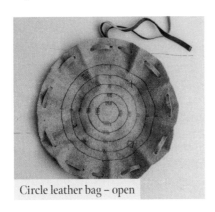
Circle leather bag – open

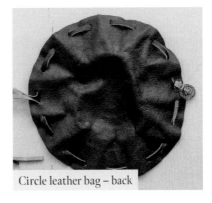
Circle leather bag – back

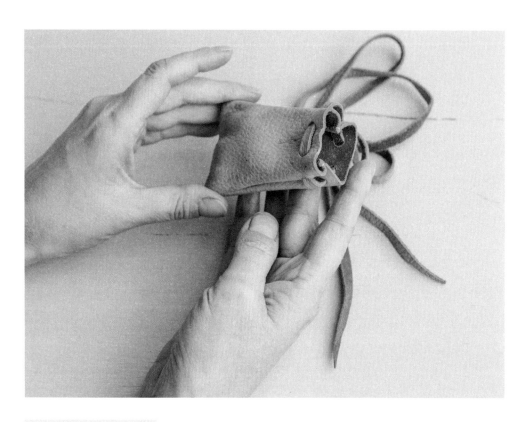

Method 3 – leather tie bag

BACK

FOLD LINE – bottom of bag

FRONT

3mm seam allowance

If you have a sewing machine, you can make another quick bag.

METHOD 3:

- *Simply cut a rectangle piece of leather twice as long as you want the bag length to be. This needs to be really soft leather. Make it as wide as you like but add an extra 3 mm on each side to allow for your seam allowance.*

- *Fold the rectangle in half with the good sides of the leather facing each other. Sew the side seams.*

- *Turn the bag the right way out and punch an even amount of holes in each side around the opening.*

- *Cut a strip of leather long enough to thread through the holes and tie around your neck if needed.*

- *Thread the leather from the back of the bag first, through the other holes and out the back again.*

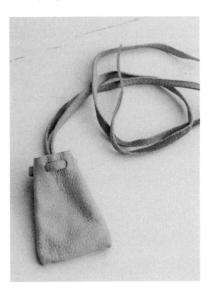

Material bag

How do you make a material bag? You can use the last pattern above but add another 1 cm seam allowance at the top of the bag.

Sew as per above, then hem the top of the bag. Fold under so it has a nice edge.

You could use eyelets for the top, or you could leave a gap in the hem at the top to thread some cord through.

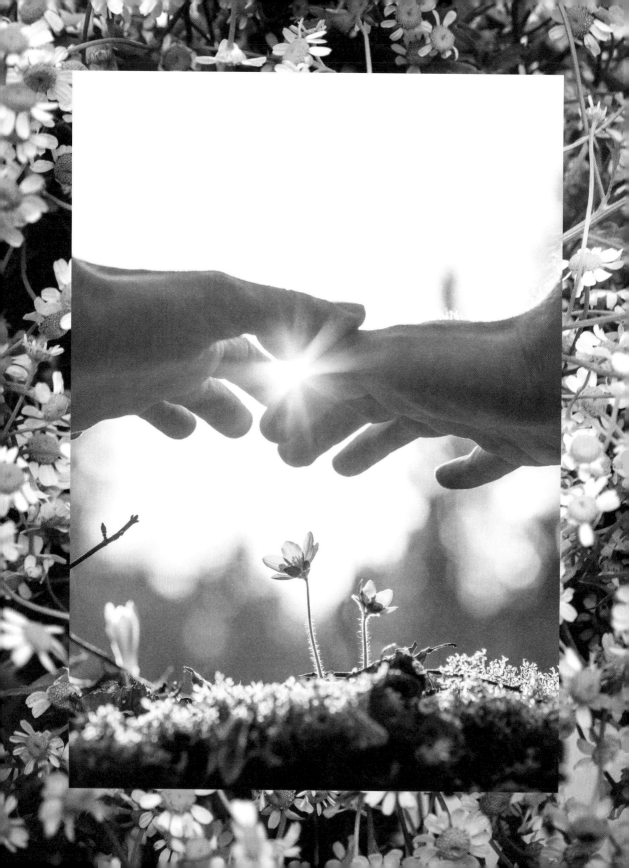

CHAPTER 8

Conclusion

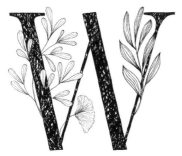 here to from here? As you can see, there are so many different kinds of Plant Spirit Medicines that can be made. The list is endless and can be overwhelming. This is where you need to sit with the plant and see how it would like to be used. If it is purely for profit, good luck with forming any kind of meaningful bond with the plant. Keep your intentions pure and be the student. Work with the plant spirits as much as you can. This is how you strengthen the connection.

Attunement

Attuning to your created Plant Spirit Medicine is very important. This is the last process of creating with the plant spirit. You might decide to perform a shamanic journey with the Plant Spirit Medicine, or simply meditate with it. There is no right or wrong way to do this, but here is an example:

1. Create your sacred space. I use sound instead of smudge to cleanse my area, so you don't have any conflicting plant spirits working with you. Tibetan bells or bowls work well, but if you don't have these just use your intention to clear your space. Make yourself comfortable, then calm and centre yourself.

2. If you have created an ingestible product, begin by ingesting a small amount. If you have created a topical product, place some on your skin where you feel guided. In the palm of your hand or inside of the wrists is a good place.

3. Ask the plant spirit to please be with you now so you may connect and learn from it.

4. Feel for any sensations in your body. Do you smell anything or hear anything? The plant spirit can make itself known to you in many ways and everyone's experience will be different. Does any imagery come to you?

5. Feel free to ask questions of the plant spirit, like:

    a. What is your message?
    b. How may I learn from you?
    c. Is there anything you need from me?
    d. How best may I use you?

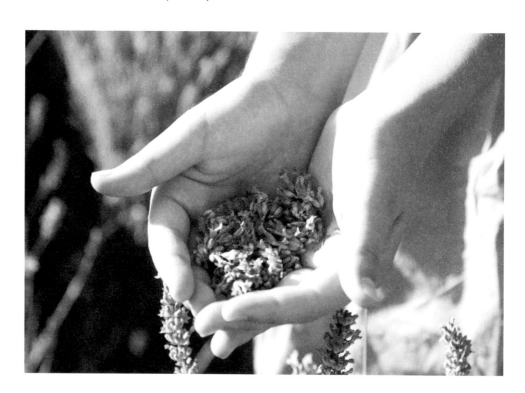

6. You might want to open your eyes and free write whatever comes to you, or draw what you see. Are any emotions or memories coming to you? Do not be concerned if you don't get much on your first sitting. These practices take time, and the more you do it the easier it becomes. I sometimes receive words or phrases as I am making the product, so every time you get any message be sure to write it down in your journal. Your journal will become an invaluable tool.

7. Once finished, be sure to thank the plant spirit and let it know that you are grateful for its teachings.

The attunement process can be done individually or in a group setting. I find this process so exciting. The information I receive is always so beautiful and gives me shivers. Over time, you will begin to feel the differences between your spirit medicines just by holding them. You might also intuitively know which ones feel right together and which ones don't.

Keep working with them, and usually when you no longer need their medicine you will forget to take or use them.

When we use our Plant Spirit Medicine what should we expect?

The answer to this will be different for everyone. Plant Spirit Medicine helps move energy within the body, whether that be emotional, spiritual or physical. So when plants have an effect on us it can come in the form of epiphanies, emotions and sometimes physical changes. Some people feel nothing at all, and some people can experience immense shifts. It also depends on the intention of the medicine, what plants were used and what application they were used in. Have faith in the process. Intention and sincerity is the key here.

Plant Spirit Medicine helps us to see our self

When we change our perception about ourselves our outer world has to change to match, because our internal environment is a reflection of our external environment and vice versa. This is how as individuals we can change the world we live in. If we all worked on healing the trauma and emotions we carry within ourselves, imagine the world we would see around us. I'm not saying that once you heal your trauma life suddenly becomes all chocolate and roses. What I'm saying is this: the world we live in is pure energy expressing itself in many ways. If we look at it in forms of dense and light energy and the law of attraction, if you are carrying dense energies you will attract dense energies. If you let go of these dense energies through letting go of stored trauma and emotions your energy being becomes lighter, attracting lighter energy to it.

Even just feeling psychologically better one day can attract beautiful experiences into your day. I know when I physically don't feel well everything seems to go wrong. Everything is an energy play. Some things we can't help but other things we can. Plants want us to be happy, they want to help. Plant Spirit Medicine is so vitally important in this day and age – and most likely always will be, as it always has been. We have untapped resources available to us that can teach, heal and guide us if we take the time to slow down and learn to make the connections.

I hope this book inspires you to make those connections.

Nicola

Even just feeling psychologically better one day can attract beautiful experiences into your day

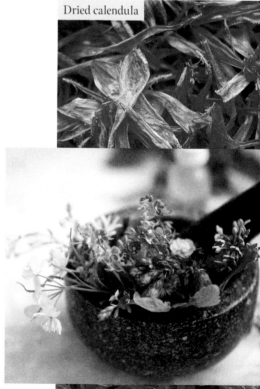

Dried calendula

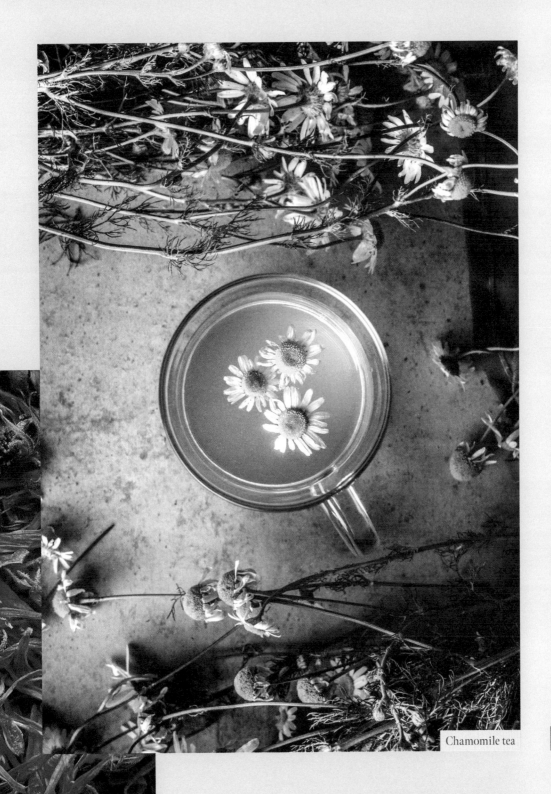

Chamomile tea

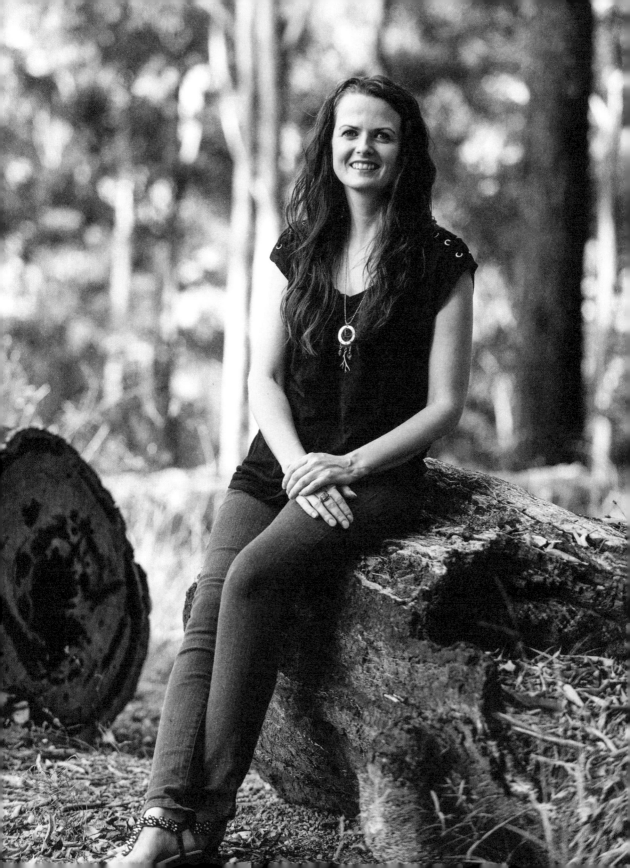

About the author

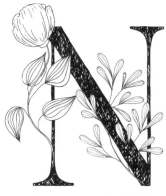

Nicola McIntosh was born in New Zealand and has lived in Australia most of her life. She resides on Tamborine Mountain nestled among the rainforest and natural surrounds. Her love of herbs started in her early 20s when she studied a Bachelor of Health Science in Western Herbal Medicine, one of the first to graduate from the newly created degree at the time. From there her love of creating natural skincare grew, and after making her own products for 20 years she felt the need to push her knowledge further. Completing a Masters of Chinese Herbal Medicine, graduating with distinction, she then pursued a Diploma of Organic Skincare Formulating.

Bringing together her years of study as well as her practice with Celtic shamanism, Nicola has brought her passion to life in her own way creating a range of herbal products alongside her oracle cards and books. Working from her home base, she formulates new products, working with all manner of herbs including some from her own garden, which allows her to understand there is so much more plants have to offer us and creating a more sustainable business. Her intention is to help others find their love for herbs and their many uses as well as finding peace for ourselves.

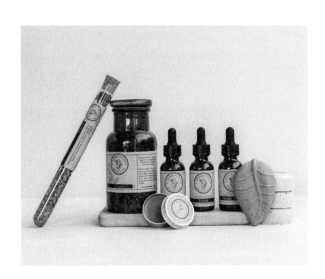

www.spiritstone.com.au

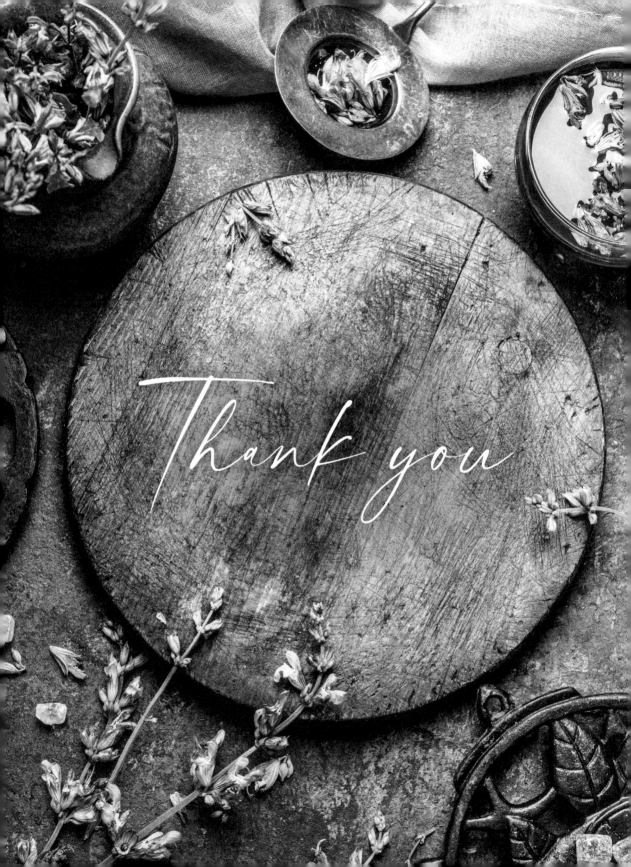

Always work

with the intent of

the highest good

for all